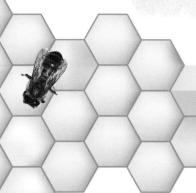

Foundations in Nursing and Health Care

Principles of Caring: A Practical Approach

Paula McGee
Series Editor: Lynne Wigens

Published in 2005 by:
Nelson Thornes Ltd
Delta Place
27 Bath Road
CHELTENHAM
GL53 7TH
United Kingdom

05 06 07 08 09 / 10 9 8 7 6 5 4 3 2 1

A catalogue record for this book is available from the British Library

ISBN 0 7487 9409 3

Illustrations by Arthur Pickering
Page make-up by Florence Production Ltd

Printed and bound in Croatia by
ZRINSKI d.d., Čakovec

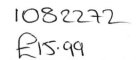

Contents

Illustrations

Preface

Nursing is a profession rooted in performance, that is to say in the undertaking of specific activities directed towards improving the health or quality of life for another person or towards alleviating that individual's suffering. None of these activities can in any meaningful way be performed alone. An individual cannot enter an empty room and say 'I am nursing in here'. Similarly, an individual cannot claim to be nursing merely by sitting and thinking about it. Nursing requires some form of activity for the benefit of another and it is in the performance of that activity that the essence of nursing becomes apparent. That essence is care. Every day and in every setting in which nursing takes place, nurses assess the need for care and then plan, implement and evaluate the impact of it. Care is so much a part of everyday nursing that it is taken for granted, but that does not make it simple or easy to perform. Care is a complex and demanding activity that requires nurses to learn a wide and sophisticated range of physical, psychological, social and intellectual skills; personal qualities, values and attributes. Nurses also have to be able to transfer that learning from one patient to the next and provide the same quality and standard of professional intervention for each one.

Care is not neutral. It is influenced by many different factors that begin with individual differences. Each individual is unique in terms of personality, preferences, likes, dislikes and even prejudices, factors that inevitably affect the ways in which people relate to one another. The type of person that the nurse is and the experiences that she or he brings to the performance of care will have an effect on relationships with patients and vice versa. Care, then, has a strong subjective element that requires nurses to become self-aware and to combine that awareness with their professional and interpersonal skills to provide nursing interventions that patients experience as care. To put it another way: two practitioners may perform exactly the same procedures, with exactly the same level of expertise but with very different attitudes and behaviour. Certain attitudes and behaviour will lead patients to experience a practitioner's performance as care. Alternatively, patients may experience a lack of care even though the performance is technically sound. The nature of care lies in the way in which it is given, rather than in what is provided.

Care is also influenced by the setting in which the nurse is practising. This can vary greatly, depending on the needs of the patients to be served. Settings for nursing care include places of work, schools and communities as well as more specialised environments such as hospitals, residential homes and prisons. The types of care required will also vary greatly and may range from performing every activity for another person to assisting them in that performance and finally to educating them about such performance in the future. Thus some forms of nursing can be very physically active as the nurse takes over from an individual all those activities that she or he would normally do unaided. Other forms of nursing are more focused on promoting independence and enabling individuals to achieve things that they previously thought impossible. Independence includes helping people to take responsibility for their own health by introducing changes in their lifestyle or by managing their health problems more effectively.

Finally, care is influenced by societal expectations. For example, current health policies reflect developments at international level to increase access to health services by making them better suited to the needs of those who use them. These developments require health professionals to relinquish outmoded ways of functioning and to adapt their practice. Learning new ways of working is not always easy but it can help to create opportunities that were previously unavailable. Nursing has benefited from such opportunities that have expanded the role and responsibilities of the profession, enabling practitioners to meet the health needs of their patients more effectively.

Care permeates the professional activities of all health practitioners, but it is in nursing that care is considered a major focus. This means that we cannot afford to take care for granted. It also means that we must not assume that others will value it if we do not explain clearly what care, in all its many forms, actually is. Those who have responsibility for calculating the cost of health services will not find it helpful if we cannot tell them clearly what we do. If we cannot tell them, and other sections of society, what we do then our work is of little account and we cannot expect to rely indefinitely on public sentiment that casts a halo over work in certain fields while ignoring it in areas that are less emotionally appealing.

Key features of the book

This book uses an interactive, dynamic approach to helping you examine the concept of care in nursing. Each chapter presents a range of activities linked to the text. Some will help you to explore certain aspects of care in detail, others will enable you to seek out additional sources or different points of view through further reading or the Internet. Wherever possible, case studies are used to help you link theoretical ideas to your own field of practice, and new terminology is explained in keyword features. You can work through each chapter alone or with a group of friends of colleagues. Each chapter closes with a short set of questions that can be used either to help you test your own learning or to formulate a quiz for use in a group.

Chapter 1 introduces you to some of the key skills that you will need not only in using this book but also in your daily practice as a nurse. These skills are concerned with your ability to adopt a questioning approach to theory and practice that will enable you to evaluate what is happening to patient care in your place of work and why. These skills are essential in modern nursing. It is no longer acceptable to do things simply because 'we have always done it this way'. As professionals, nurses need to look carefully at the evidence on which they base their practice and determine whether it is sufficiently robust to warrant continued use or whether more recent and better evidence indicates that it is time to change. Asking questions rather than accepting the status quo is the foundation of critical practice skills. Chapter 1 expands on these, helping you to think about the types of questions you might ask. The chapter then helps you to relate your new skills to an examination of care as a theoretical concept and, in particular, as a focus for nursing work. By the end this chapter you should be able to begin to evaluate any new set of theoretical ideas.

Chapter 2 presents the foundations of modern professional nursing, which is focused around four key concepts: the person, health, the environment and nursing. Each of these terms is explained and the chapter then enables you to examine one of these concepts in detail (the person) by drawing on research into patients' experiences of receiving care. Case studies are included to help you gain an understanding of what it is that patients regard as care and being cared for. These case studies will help you to see that, while technical skill and professional knowledge are important, what matters more to patients is the attitudes and behaviour of professionals. By the end of this chapter you will have gained an understanding of what it is like to feel cared for by a nurse.

Chapter 3 helps you to look at the second aspect of nursing: nursing itself. In particular, this chapter enables you to examine care from the nurse's perspective beginning with the nursing process, the cyclical framework that forms the basis of the care we give to patients. Inherent in this framework are specific activities such as assessment, nursing diagnosis and goal setting. Each of these activities is discussed and exercises are included to help you broaden your knowledge. The application of the nursing process is influenced by whatever theory nurses use to underpin their work. There is no single theory that will suit every setting in which nursing care takes place because each nurse theorist presents different ideas about the nature of care. Chapter 3 uses case studies are used to help you explore the ways in which different nursing theories can influence the use of the nursing process with patients. Further exercises then help you to critically examine the way in which theory informs the application of the nursing process in your own place of work. By the end of this chapter you will have gained a deeper understanding of the theoretical basis for nursing practice and the ways in which the use of theory impacts on the application of the nursing process.

Chapter 4 continues the focus on the second aspect of nursing by enabling you to examine the care within the context of secondary care, that is, care in a hospital setting. Case studies are used to help you draw on different nursing theories in an exploration of the diversity of nursing practice through two concepts: direct and indirect care. In considering each of these you will see that nurses working directly with patients form therapeutic relationships with their patients. In these relationships nurses adopt a multiplicity of roles depending on both the needs of the individuals for whom they are caring and the personal characteristics of the nurse concerned. This chapter will help you to appreciate that working directly with patients requires an awareness of the self, of how we as individuals appear to others, and an honest appraisal of our strengths and weaknesses. Case studies in this chapter will also help you to see that nurses who do not work directly with patients all the time, or perhaps not at all, nevertheless have important roles and responsibilities in providing care. By the end of this chapter you will have gained an understanding of nursing roles in a hospital setting and an appreciation of the professional accountability that underpins the provision of nursing care in hospitals.

Chapter 5 provides an opportunity for you to look at the two remaining aspects of nursing, the environment and health, within the context of primary care. These two aspects are brought together in this chapter because they are closely related. Examining ideas about health leads inevitably to a study of the environments in which people live, work and participate in leisure activities or receive an education. The interplay between health and the environment means that each acts upon the other. Thus separating them is not necessarily helpful. Examining both within primary care is appropriate because the majority of patients who receive some form of nursing care are not in hospital and, for many individuals, the use of primary care services represents their only contact with the NHS. Various exercises and case studies are used to introduce you to recent developments in primary that are intended to empower those with long term health problems to become more independent of day-to-day professional support. These developments are also aimed at helping professionals to work in new ways that enable them to provide better support for such patients, anticipate, and take a proactive role in preventing, the development of problems. By the end of this chapter you will have gained an understanding of the importance of health and the environment in nursing and of current approaches to the management of long term health problems in primary care settings.

Chapter 6 is based on the recognition that Britain is a diverse society in which members of many different cultures and traditions co-exist. As this chapter makes clear, the concept of care is universal but differences in cultural values, beliefs and traditions influence its expression. Thus what is valued as care in one culture may be regarded quite negatively in another. This chapter helps you to explore the ways in which culture impacts on the provision of nursing care. Exercises and case studies will help you to see differences in how people think about themselves as people, what they believe causes illness, the interrelationship between themselves and the environment and the implications of this for the provision of care using the nursing process. In particular, this chapter revisits the idea that professionals need to adapt to new ways of working that was introduced in chapter 5. In chapter 6, this idea is developed further in terms of laying aside professional dominance and engaging with patients on a more equal footing. This means that care should be negotiated with the patient rather than simply delivered in a way that may or may not be suitable. By the end of this chapter you will have gained insight into the ways in which culture affects the provision and experience of care and developed understanding of appropriate strategies that will help you to care for patients.

Chapter 7 introduces a second major influence on care, namely the Internet. The introduction of Internet access into the workplace has enabled professionals to gain easy access to a wide range of resources and has provided opportunities both to share good practice and to learn from others. Patients too have benefited from access to the Internet, which enables them to become much better informed, use the net to promote self-care and self-help and to find out about ways in which they can improve their health. These benefits to patients have brought changes in the ways in which patients relate to professionals. Patients are not longer willing to comply with instructions simply because the doctor or the nurse has told them what to do. Patients now expect to be involved in decision-making about their care and this chapter helps you consider current moves to encourage this trend through the introduction of the expert patient scheme. However, as far as the Internet is concerned, the quality and accuracy of material available on the Internet varies greatly and professionals have a responsibility to provide guidance for patients about the appropriateness of particular websites. By the end of this chapter you will have learned how to direct your questioning approach and evaluative skills towards the business of reviewing web sites related to your field of practice.

Chapter 8 addresses a third major factor that influences care: multi-professional working. Other health professions besides nursing are experiencing change as part of the emphasis on improving both the accessibility and the quality of services. This chapter enables you to explore, through exercises and case studies, the healthcare context in which professionals are required to work more closely together. Effective multi-professional collaboration is essential in ensuring that patients receive services that are coherent, because all the parties involved actively contribute to an agreed plan of action that is regularly reviewed, rather than a disjointed effort in which no one knows what anyone else is doing. This multi-professional approach is particularly important in a modern health service where no one profession or individual practitioner can meet the needs of all patients, particularly those with complex or enduring heath problems. Teamwork is essential particularly given the increasing impact of new technologies in almost every aspect of health care. Examples include keyhole surgery, the use of ultrasound and new pharmaceutical products. By the end of this chapter you will have examined the key issues in providing nursing care within a multi-professional context.

Chapter 9 helps you to explore your own development as a provider of nursing care through case studies and exercises. Learning to care requires a synthesis of theoretical and practical knowledge based on exposure to health problems and the needs of patients. Such exposure creates what Benner (1984) termed paradigm cases, situations that challenge the individual's view of the status quo and enable that person to adapt and change their practice to meet the particular requirements of the situation. Developing such flexibility takes the nurse through a series of stages, beginning as a novice who has limited knowledge and skill and who thus depends on context free rules to guide performance. Gradually the nurse progresses to become a proficient practitioner who is able to view patients holistically and adopt a flexible approach to providing care while relying to some extent on rules to guide practice (Benner 1984). Such proficiency is, however, not the end of the story. The proficient practitioner still has much to learn in order to become an expert who no longer depends on rules and whose extensive experience facilitates an accurate perception of what is truly important in each situation and a subsequent fluid and flexible approach to care (Benner 1984). The expert nurse, therefore, uses a sophisticated blend of theoretical and practical knowledge combined with a wide range of paradigm cases. Such expertise reflects a 'state of professional maturity in which the individual demonstrates a level of integrated knowledge, skill and competence that challenges the accepted boundaries of practice and pioneers new developments in healthcare' (McGee and Castledine 2003 p. 24).

Inherent in becoming an expert is the ability to engage in a critical approach to practice. Chapter 9 revisits the key skills introduced at the beginning of this book and provides exercises that will help you to apply these skills to the appraisal of evidence that provides a rationale for care. This chapter helps you to understand the different levels of evidence available in health care and how these may be evaluated to enable you to feel confident in selecting the most robust as a basis for your practice. As this chapter demonstrates, there is no clear agreement about what constitutes sound evidence because health care is constantly changing and no two patients are quite the same. Expert practitioners must, therefore, be able to make ethical decisions about what is best, given the particular circumstances and resources available. By the end of this chapter you will have learned how to use your questioning approach and evaluative skill in the provision of evidence-based care.

Chapter 10 helps you to contextualise current influences on nursing care by examining current health policies. These policies are intended to improve the quality and standards of health services. Moreover, services are required to reflect the needs of local populations. Service providers must ensure that patients have equity in accessing services irrespective of any particular characteristics. This chapter begins by explaining the background from which current policies emerged and, in particular, the NHS Plan (DOH 2000) that provided the basis for radical reform. Various aspects of reform are then examined in more detail including the role of the National Institute for Clinical Excellence (NICE), National Service frameworks and clinical governance. Each of these is discussed in detail and several exercises are included to help you relate these reforms to your field. By the end of this chapter you will have gained an understanding of the key elements of current health policies and how these impact on your field of practice.

Chapter 11 brings the book to a close by summarising the key points made about care and setting an agenda for the future. Care is the underlying principle on which nursing activities are based. Providing nursing care in a modern health service is a complex and demanding activity that requires the distillation of a wide range of knowledge and skill into appropriate and humane interventions that improve health and alleviate suffering. The diversity of expertise and the individuality of each patient means that there is still much to explore and to learn about care. This chapter identifies three key areas in which research is required to expand our understanding of what patients experience as care and how we can best balance the technological possibilities with human needs. The nurse's therapeutic use of self is pivotal in the provision of holistic care within a health service that is structured around the wishes and preferences of its clients as opposed to those of its providers. This radical shift in emphasis has not been attempted before and has the potential to alter significantly the ways in which patients and nurses relate to one another. We shall need research to examine the new form of therapeutic relationship and identify ways in which nurses can best harness the resources available to provide care. Patients too will have to learn new ways of dealing with their health problems and become more independent of professional support. Whatever happens, as this chapter points out, professionals will have to find new ways of working while at the same time avoiding making matters worse. Focusing on care as an underlying principle for nursing activities will help to ensure that the well being of patients remains the paramount concern.

References

Benner, P. (1984) *From Novice to Expert. Excellence and Power in Clinical Nursing*. Menlo Park CA, Addison-Wesley.

McGee, P. and Castledine, G. (2003) 'A definition of advanced practice for the UK', Chapter 3 P. McGee and G. Castledine (eds) *Advanced Practice,* 2nd edn. Oxford, Blackwell Science, pp. 17-32.

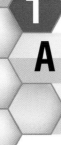

1

A critical approach to care in nursing

Learning outcomes

By the end of this chapter you should be able to:

- identify and begin to practise the skills needed to think critically about theoretical ideas;
- apply these skills in examining the concept of care in nursing;
- begin to relate your knowledge about nursing care to your practice;
- identify some of the factors that may influence the delivery of nursing care.

Introduction

Professional nursing takes place within a cyclical process in which each patient's health problems are identified through systematic assessment, suitable interventions are planned and implemented and subsequent outcomes are evaluated. This process takes into account the individual's lifestyle and circumstances and may occur within the context of that person's home, workplace or community – or in a hospital setting. Nursing is thus a diverse profession in which the work undertaken in one place may be totally at variance with that performed in another and yet the same principles underpin the approach to patients in both circumstances. Inherent in this process is the concept of care, which forms the core around which nursing takes place. This concept is complex and influenced not only by individual needs and circumstances but also by a wide range of other factors such as the expectations of society, current health policy and professional standards.

This chapter helps you to examine this concept of care through a series of exercises. These begin with a discussion about the need for critical thinking, one of the key skills needed in nursing generally but especially important when considering a topic about which there are numerous theories that may at times appear to contradict one another. None is of any use to practitioners unless they can relate the ideas presented to the realities of nursing practice. Consequently, the approach to critical thinking introduced in this chapter is intended not only to help you adopt a questioning approach to the theoretical study of care but also to consider the extent to which theory can be applied.

Keywords

Critical approach
This term means that we do
not accept the status quo
simply because that is how
things are done. We ask
questions, take a flexible
approach to the examination of
practice from different
perspectives and assess the
quality of evidence available to
inform the development of best
practice.

Thinking critically

The complex nature of care means that there is no single definition
or theoretical perspective that encompasses every aspect of it. Each
theorist or researcher provides us with a particular point of view that
may or may not be appropriate for an individual practice setting. You
therefore need to adopt a **critical approach** to thinking about
nursing theory and practice in order to determine the usefulness
and applicability of specific ideas about care, evaluate the extent to
which practice needs to change and clarify ways in which patients
will benefit as a result. Finally, a critical approach to practice helps
to develop and evaluate strategies for improving care. This approach
is not about criticising in the everyday sense of the word. A critical
approach to practice is about thinking, how we think and what we
think about.

Thinking is a complex activity that we tend to take for granted
and yet it involves several different mental activities. De Bono
(2004) argues that the focus of our thinking activities changes as we
get older. Up to the age of about five we tend to be concerned with
why things are as they are. Between the ages of six and about
twelve, we tend to concentrate on challenging things as they are by
asking *why not?* For example, why not try something new? Why not
try things a different way? As we move towards adulthood we start to
lose that curiosity and start to accept that things are as they are
because that is how the world is. Adams (2002) makes similar points
about the way we react to new ideas. He argues that when we are
born we accept everything that is in the world as normal. Anything
new that comes along before we reach our thirtieth birthday we tend
to regard as exciting and may even be able to make a career out of it.
After our thirtieth birthday, we start to become cautious and view
new ideas with scepticism or even resist them altogether (Adams
2002). Both Adams and De Bono are drawing our attention to the
ways in which our thinking can become rigid and narrow in focus,
preventing us from examining an idea or situation clearly. To help
prevent this De Bono (2004) developed his Six Thinking Hats
theory that facilitates a flexible and logical approach to thinking
(see Figure 1.1).

This theory is based on the notion that thinking requires the
consideration of six elements. De Bono has used the theory in
teaching children to think and in that context coloured hats
provided a way of structuring exercises. The colour of each hat
refers to a different aspect of thinking. In thinking with the red hat
we examine our feelings about the subject. In challenging situations
it is easy to let emotions guide our actions but this theory requires

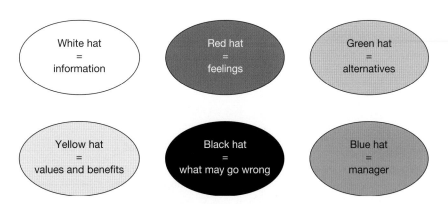

Figure 1.1 *De Bono's Six Thinking Hats*

us to look at our feelings and lay them on one side while we look at the matter from other perspectives. Thinking with the yellow hat helps us to consider the positive sides of the situation – the values and benefits that may already be there or that may arise from a proposed change. Thinking with the green hat asks us to consider alternatives to the current situation or proposed course of action so that we examine a range of possibilities. Thinking with the black hat helps us to think about what may go wrong if we either maintain the situation as it is or seek to change it. Thinking with the white hat helps to identify the information we need in order to move forward. These hats do not have to be used in any particular order but, in allowing an equal amount of time for thinking with each one, we are likely to reach a balanced view that enables us to make sound decisions. Thinking with the blue hat then provides us with an opportunity to consider what we should do next and make a plan.

Theory into Practice

Select a practice-based topic that has recently been discussed in your place of work. How might an understanding of the Six Thinking Hats theory help you and your colleagues to address this topic?

Thinking about thinking and how we think helps us to consider the next step: what we think about. In nursing, the term *critical approach* is used to refer to thinking about practice. Nurses are encouraged to examine their practice, and determine whether it is informed by theory or research rather than custom, routine or convenience. Practice must have an up-to-date evidence base and at the same time meet the specific needs of each individual patient. Thus nurses are continually striving to evaluate and improve their practice. This critical approach requires three

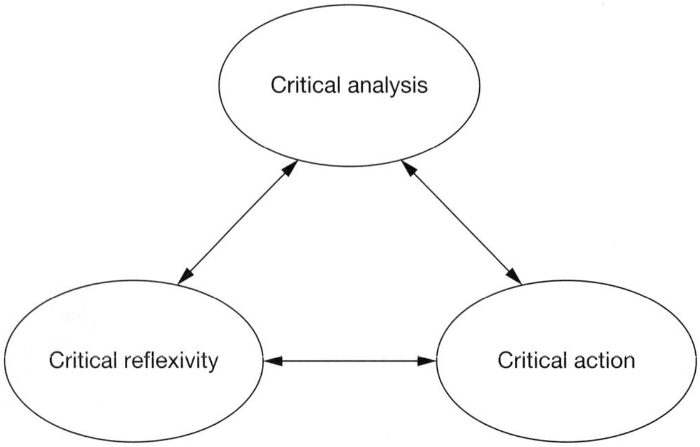

Figure 1.2 *Elements of a critical approach to practice*

elements: *critical analysis, critical action* and *critical reflexivity* (see Figure 1.2). These three elements inform each other in a dynamic appraisal of practice and ideas. This critical approach to practice is a key component of this book and the following exercise will help you begin to develop your own skills in this area (Brechin 2000).

Over to you

Analyse a nursing theory with which you are familiar or analyse a research-based article about practice in the professional nursing journal that you usually read. Try to answer the following questions:

1 What is the background of the writer?
2 What information is provided about the writer?
3 Is this person writing from the perspective of nursing or putting forward information or ideas from another discipline such as sociology or psychology?
4 How was the theory/research developed?
5 Has the writer drawn on other established theories or research but made clear how his/her ideas differ from what has gone before?
6 What is the aim of the theory/research: is it to describe something that happens, explain why something happens or predict what may happen?
7 Is the theory/research clearly explained?
8 Have the ideas it proposes been piloted or tested in practice settings?
9 How was this done and what were the outcomes?
10 What does the theory/ research say?

Make a list summarising the key points. Use these to explain the theory/research to someone else.

11 What does this theory/research contribute to practice in my field?

Only you can answer this but it is worth considering here the relevance of the theory/research and your own evaluation of current practice in your particular setting. In addition, try to find out whether anyone else has critically evaluated or tried to apply the theory/research and identify the outcomes obtained.

12 Does this theory/research provide something that my patients want or need?

The best way to ascertain what patients want is to ask them. Find out how your organisation accesses the views of patients and what in-house procedures will enable you to ask them about the changes that may be needed if you are to implement this theory/research.

13 How feasible would it be to implement this theory/research?

In considering this question try to make a list of the specific criteria for successful application of this theory/research in your practice setting. Make a second list of possible obstacles. These may be physical, psychological, legal or even social. For example, physical obstacles may include the geographical layout of a particular hospital ward that may favour certain ways of organising work. Psychological obstacles could include people's resistance to change or perhaps patients' reactions to interventions that cause unpleasant side effects. Theory/research developed in another country may not be consistent with legal nursing practice in your setting. Social obstacles can be generated by the introduction of change. For example, work-based teams may have to be split up. In addition you may need to consider whether you have sufficient information to implement the theory/research and whether staff would require further training to develop or adapt their skills. None of the obstacles is intended to be seen as an excuse for inaction if the theory or research really has the potential to help bring about improvements, but each possibility must be carefully considered. Implementing change requires careful planning, which includes strategies for dealing with obstacles.

Reflective activity

In light of the 'Over to you' exercise above, consider the following questions:

● How can I bring about change?
● What are my strengths and what are my weaknesses?
● What am I trying to achieve?
● How can I communicate this to others effectively?
● Am I receptive to their views and opinions and willing to modify my ideas?
● Who do I need to convince?
● How will I know whether I have been successful?

⊶ₙ *Keywords*

Critical analysis
The ability to review information from different angles or view points presented.

Critical action
The ability to act or put actions into place in the most appropriate way.

Critical reflexivity
The ability to think about a situation or action that has occurred using all of the evidence presented.

Critical analysis is an open-minded, reflective and questioning attitude that is receptive to new ideas. The key skills needed are the ability to analyse and evaluate new information, and the ability to make decisions about the extent to which such information is credible and likely to make a useful contribution to practice. Being critical in this context is about recognising that there is more than one point of view and about using your professional knowledge to determine the usefulness and applicability of new ideas to your particular practice settings. **Critical action** involves the ability to evaluate existing practice in the light of new information and determine the feasibility of introducing change. Key skills required include the ability to identify the criteria for success and the likely obstacles, planning the introduction of change and evaluating progress. **Critical reflexivity** requires each practitioner to develop self-awareness through the use of reflective skills. Reflection may be undertaken as a personal activity to examine particular events or experiences. However, individualistic reflection has limited learning potential. Developing self-awareness is dependent on dialogue with others, interacting, discussing ideas and reviewing the feedback obtained. Not only does this help to refine and modify ideas but it also enables individuals to review and develop their interpersonal competence. This is crucial to critical reflexivity in which the key skills revolve around the ability to interact with others and negotiate with them, particularly those who may have doubts or disagree with what is proposed. Empowering others to take ownership of new ideas and incorporate these into their practice requires high levels of interpersonal skill that are critical to the success of any new venture (Brechin 2000; Eby 2000).

Key points Top tips

- Nursing is a diverse profession encompassing a wide range of settings, knowledge and skills.
- The core or focal point of nursing is the provision of care to patients.
- The type of care provided depends on the individuals concerned and the situation.
- The provision of care is influenced by factors outside the situation.
- Successful and effective care is dependent on the way in which nurses think about their practice.
- A critical approach to practice enables nurses to evaluate and improve their practice.
- A critical approach has three elements: critical analysis, critical action and critical reflexivity.

Defining care

Meanings of 'care'

Are there any links or relationships between the points you have written down?

In Figure 1.3 we can see that care somehow involves other people, how they treat us and how, in return, we treat them. Those who care about us behave in certain ways towards us. These ways may be difficult to define because, quite often, we do not think consciously about how people treat us until they do so in a negative way. We have all encountered others who we think *don't care*, *couldn't care less*, *are uncaring* because of the way they have treated us.

First of all, care is *intentional*, that is to say that it is consciously directed towards others. We care *for* or *about* another person, and

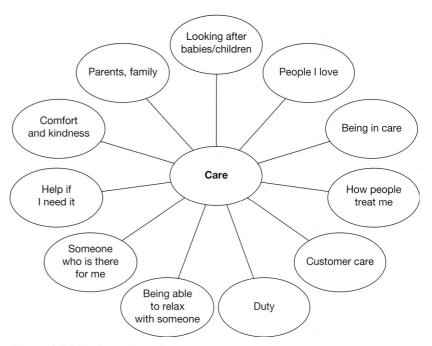

Figure 1.3 *Meanings of 'care'*

thus at least two people are required for care to take place: the giver and the receiver (Edwards 2001). Intentional care in nursing is deliberately directed towards improving the situation of another, for example by relieving pain or discomfort, cleaning, feeding or sharing an experience with that person. Care is therefore *relational*, requiring 'actions that help, support or facilitate another individual. Those actions may have physical, psychological, social, environmental or cultural dimensions' (Leininger 1984 p. 3) and, in nursing, serve to emphasise the high value that nurses tend to place on doing things with or for patients. Direct activity with patients, such as carrying out total patient care, working as a primary nurse, or working with others to help them develop new skills, particularly in the management of those with complex or unusual needs, is valued above other work because it is only through direct engagement with patients that the purpose of nursing 'to promote health, healing and normal growth and development; to prevent illness; and, when people become ill, to minimise distress and suffering and to enable them to understand and cope with their disease, its treatment and consequences' can be enacted (Royal College of Nursing (RCN) 2002 p. 2). Without that engagement, the whole idea of nursing is meaningless. Like dance, drama and other performance-based professions, nursing only comes to life through performance. Sustained engagement in direct work with patients in a range of settings and with different client groups is now essential for the development of a practice-based career in which extensive experience is synthesised with theoretical knowledge and then applied to practice (Oberle and Allen 2001). Such synthesis, plus regular and substantial practice, are mandatory components of many senior and advanced roles, such as those of nurse consultants, whose posts were introduced with the intention of providing practice-based leadership and require post holders to spend the greater part of their working time in practice (Department of Health (DOH) 1999; National Health Service Executive (NHSE) 1999).

Alongside this relationship between care and others are the concepts of responsibility and expectation. Parents are expected to care for their children: to treat them in certain ways that will ensure healthy and happy physical, psychological and social growth into adulthood. Failure to care or lack of care by parents attracts censure. We may have expectations of family and perhaps friends to provide social and emotional help, particularly when we are in difficulties, and we feel we have a responsibility to return that help when it is needed. All of this giving and receiving is bound up with our feelings: feelings of gratitude or pleasure when we receive or give care and our feelings of rejection or pain when care is not forthcoming. Care is, therefore, *ontological*, that is to say it is part of our experience of being in the world. In our early lives we are the recipients of care from others. This teaches us that, in order to live in the world, we have to interact with others to maintain our own well-being and they in turn must interact with us. Care is an integral part of what it is to be a human being (Edwards 2001). Care requires us to set priorities as a basis for giving and receiving in a mutually beneficial way. Too much attention to the self will militate against engagement with others and what we receive from them. Engaging with others brings rewards that outweigh attention to the self. Thus other people are worth investing in. Other people are valuable because care 'sets up the condition that something or someone outside the person matters and creates personal concerns' that provide motivation and directions for the self (Benner and Wrubel 1989 p. 1). This ontological aspect of care is so ingrained in us that we may take it for granted or even cease to think about it. In such circumstances, care lacks intentionality and is either performed without thinking or assumed to exist in situations where it may or may not be actually present.

To explain that statement further, our society places expectations and responsibilities on suppliers and vendors to sell us goods and services of appropriate quality that do no harm to people and that are fit for the intended purpose. Commercial companies recognise that looking after their customers, customer care, is an important part of their business. However, most of us have experienced the frustrations that arise when some appliance breaks down and care seems to be noticeably lacking when we try to seek help or redress. We expect care, assume that it is present and, when it is not forthcoming, tend to respond emotionally. In reality, from the commercial point of view we are simply engaging in another business transaction.

Similarly, society places responsibilities on, and has expectations of, those whose job it is to provide services for particular groups of people. The sick, the disabled or those with mental health problems or learning difficulties are deemed by society to be vulnerable because of their dependence on others. Those whose work requires them to provide services to members of these groups are expected to treat them in ways that uphold individual dignity. Lack of care in these situations also tends to evoke emotional responses because it is taken for granted that the people concerned can be trusted. Thus, care has a strong emotional dimension in that when we talk about caring we are really talking about our feelings (Smith 1992).

However, looking again at the links and relationships in our brainstorming (Figure 1.3) we can see that care is also about dependence and action, about doing something for another that they cannot do for themselves. In the context of family and friends, caring for others requires physical, psychological and social effort. In the commercial sphere, people are employed to undertake care work, work that usually involves direct contact with the public and that draws upon well-developed interpersonal skills to field complaints, sort out problems and ensure customer satisfaction. In health and social care people are employed to look after others who are in some way dependent on their services. Like workers in the commercial sector, their work requires direct contact with their clients, sometimes for long periods of time and frequently in emotionally charged situations. Unlike workers in the commercial sector, those in health and social care are likely to have patients or clients who are highly dependent on them and for whom the delivery of care requires the level of intimacy normally shared among close family members or friends. Care is work, a particular type of work, that requires not only physical but also mental and emotional strength and effort. It is emotional labour (Smith 1992 p. 7), 'the induction or suppression of (our) feeling to sustain an outward appearance that produces in others a sense of being cared for in a convivial place'. It does not come easily or naturally. We have to learn from others how to care because it is through being cared for that we are able best to care for others. Those employed in care work face particular challenges and 'have to work emotionally on themselves in order to appear to care, irrespective of how they personally feel about themselves, individual patients, their conditions and circumstances. They can also be taught to manage their feelings more effectively' (Smith 1992 p. 136).

Arguments for Smith's statement

Care can be emotionally draining and tiring. It can be hard to empathise with another person and relate to their difficulties. We may not necessarily know what to say or do for the best and we need others to show us. Sometimes, the people we are caring for are not people we particularly like, and we have to make an effort to do what is needed.

Arguments against Smith's statement

As professionals we have a responsibility to provide care irrespective of any distinguishing characteristics that the patient may have. We have a duty of care that exists independently of any feelings we may have. While the circumstances of some patients do evoke feelings in us, this does not occur with everyone.

Key points Top tips

- There is no single definition of care.
- Care is directed towards other people; it is based on giving to others and receiving from them.
- Care has physical, psychological, social, environmental, emotional and cultural dimensions.
- Care is a performing art like dance or drama.
- We have to learn how to care for other people.
- We take care for granted but failure to care invites censure.
- Care is a type of work that requires physical, emotional and psychological effort.
- The professional provision of care carries responsibility.

Care as a focus for nursing

Several theories of nursing have placed care at the centre of nursing work. The most noted of these is Leininger (1984 p. 3) who states that care is 'the essence of and unifying *intellectual and practical* dimension of professional nursing', which differentiates nursing from other professions, notably medicine:

> Caring refers to the *direct* (or indirect) *nurturant* and *skilful* activities, *processes and decisions* related to assisting people in such a manner that reflects behavioural attributes which are *empathetic, supportive, compassionate, protective, succorant, educational* and others dependent on the needs, problems, values and goals of the individual or group being assisted.
>
> (My emphasis, Leininger 1984)

She argues that care refers to actions that help, support or facilitate another individual or group to relieve or improve their situation. These actions may involve physical activities, but there are also psychological, social, environmental and cultural dimensions to providing care (Leininger 1984). Leininger identifies three forms of care: folk, professional and nursing. Folk or lay care is based on knowledge, skill and tradition from within a specific culture. It enables members of particular cultures to improve health and provide help and support to those who are ill, disabled or dying (Leininger and McFarland 2002). In her view, this type of care contrasts with professional care, which she defines as that provided by Western health care services in which knowledge and skills originate from scientific and technological sources. Like folk care, professional care is directed towards helping others to maintain or improve their health or recover from illness, but it comes from a different perspective. Nursing care draws on both professional and folk care as well as its own knowledge base in order to provide care (Leininger and McFarland 2002).

Emphasis on care as an important element in nursing is also to be found in the work of other nurse theorists. For example, Watson (1999 pp. 27–8) states that care is a major focus for nursing 'not only because of the *dynamic human-to-human transactions*, but because of the requirements of *knowledge, commitment* and *human values* and because of the *personal, social and moral engagement* of the nurse in time and space'. In her view care is the moral ideal of nursing 'whereby the end is protection, enhancement and the preservation of human dignity' (my emphasis, Watson 1999 p. 29).

Reflective activity

Think of a patient you have nursed. To what extent did the nursing care given to that person reflect what Leininger and Watson are saying?

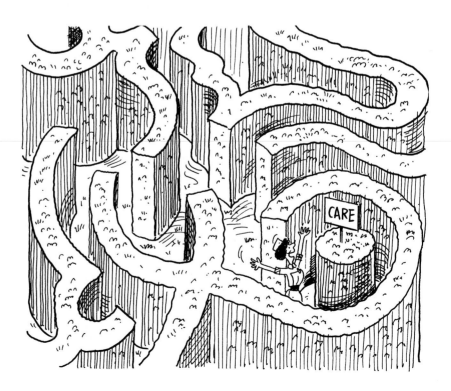

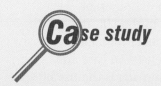
Case study

Hyacinth Williams is 57 years old. She and her husband run a newsagent and general store that is open between 6.30 a.m. and 7 p.m. every day except Sunday. Five years ago, Hyacinth began to experience periods of extreme thirst. She felt tired all the time and complained of giddiness. She also had some numbness in her toes. She was diagnosed as having diabetes, which she manages through a combination of dietary control and regular injections of insulin. At times she finds controlling her blood sugar levels a difficult and frustrating business, although she usually manages fairly well. Earlier this week her granddaughter came home early from school because Hyacinth was not feeling well and yesterday Hyacinth had a sore throat and a headache. She felt unwell but not ill enough, in her opinion, to go to the doctor. Throughout the day she became increasingly thirsty. She decided to take a short nap during the afternoon in the hope that things would improve with rest. Her family were alarmed when they could not rouse her and she was admitted to hospital in a hyperglycaemic coma.

Analysis using Leininger's views

Hyacinth has been admitted as an emergency. She will require the direct administration of practical and skilful nursing activities that are based on sound technological and scientific knowledge about how best to stabilise her blood sugar and insulin levels. She will need support and empathy as she may be very frightened as she regains consciousness and fear that she may die. She will require protective nursing activities to prevent any further harm while she is unable to care for herself. When she has recovered from her hyperglycaemia, she will need educational nursing activities that take account of her cultural beliefs and values in order to prevent a recurrence.

Analysis using Watson's views

Hyacinth has been admitted as an emergency and might die if she is not treated quickly and appropriately. Caring requires a commitment to action based on knowledge of what is appropriate. It requires individuals motivated and able to perform whatever is required. Caring for this patient is a moral activity that is based on valuing her as a person, recognising her need for care, acting on the recognition and bringing about an appropriate change.

In analysing these two theoretical positions we can see that both theorists express similar ideas about care as a central focus for nursing. Both Leininger and Watson see nursing care as our behaviour towards and involvement with others based on knowledge, skill and commitment. Leininger provides more detail about the nature of that behaviour and involvement while Watson provides more of the moral and ethical reasons for activities.

Care gives a focus for nursing activities. It helps to define what it is that nurses do in a way that can be explained to others. While there is evidence that skilled nursing care makes a difference (Needleman *et al.* 2002) it can be difficult to express clearly what that difference is. If we are unable to state clearly what we are doing when we nurse, then we cannot expect others to value or pay for it or to want to join the profession. Consequently, a definition of nursing that is meaningful to others is essential. In the UK, the Royal College of Nursing has supported the argument for a clear definition of nursing. The College's definition focuses on care and the purposes towards which it can be directed: 'nursing is the use of clinical judgement and the provision of care to enable people to promote, improve, maintain or recover health or, when death is inevitable, to die peacefully' (RCN 2002).

However, in appropriating care, nursing places itself in an adversarial position regarding other health professions. Kleinman (1988 p. 253), for example, states that the purpose of medicine is 'both the control of the disease process and care for the illness experience'. In other words, the practice of medicine should be patient-focused and directed as much towards care as attempted cure. Care in this context is about listening to patients, recognising them as people and treating them rather than their diseases. If we accept Kleinman's argument, then nursing cannot claim to have a monopoly on care, but nurses may be able to argue that the type of care provided by doctors differs from that of nurses or that the emphasis on care is different within the two professions.

Key points Top tips

- Several nurse theorists see care as a focal point for nursing.
- One example is Leininger, one of the key theorists in care in nursing, who identifies three forms of care: folk, professional and lay.
- A second example is Watson, who sees care as a moral ideal for nursing.
- Clarifying the concept of care is essential in nursing to help others, especially those in power, to understand what nurses do.
- The Royal College of Nursing has developed a definition of nursing.
- Care may be the focal point of nursing, but this does not automatically imply a monopoly: members of other professions may also regard their role as one of providing care.

Influences on care in nursing

The concept of care provides a vehicle for explaining to others, both within and outside the profession, what it is that nurses do. However, providing care is a process of negotiation between what the profession can be held responsible for, what it can provide and what others expect. Consequently, the provision of nursing care is influenced by many different factors.

Reflec**Reflective activity**

Think about what factors may have influenced the nature of care that you have given to patients.

Figure 1.4 provides a summary of the points that you may have identified. First are social factors. Changes in UK society have challenged the traditional hegemony of professional groups. People now want and have the right to be involved in decisions about their health and to challenge professional opinion. Access to other sources of information, especially via the Internet, enables patients today to find out more about their condition and treatment options than any previous generation. Consequently, professionals now have a much greater responsibility to explain to patients the courses of action available and to help individuals to make informed and appropriate choices that suit their circumstances (Hardey 2001; DOH 2003). The impact of television dramas such as *Casualty* help to promote public understanding of nursing roles and the types of work in which they are engaged. They may also influence public expectations about care. Finally, the UK is a multicultural and multiracial society. Leininger (Leininger and McFarland 2002) was the first nurse theorist, to recognise that culture has a profound impact on care. Her research identified that, while caring for others is a universal phenomenon found in all societies, what is perceived as care varies from one to another. Effective care

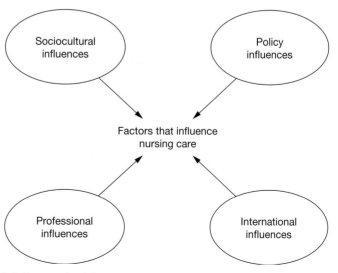

Figure 1.4 *Factors that influence nursing care*

is care that is in tune with people's cultural values and beliefs (McGee 2000).

Second are international factors that have influenced both UK law and the practice of nursing. For example, the European Charter of Human Rights (www.europarl.eu.int/charter) makes plain that every individual has the right to make decisions about himself or herself without pressure from others. Each individual also has the right not to be subjected to unwanted interference. Special groups such as the elderly, those with disabilities and children also have specific rights to ensure that they are treated as full members of society. Other rights deal with issues such as data protection and freedom from discrimination. A second document on human rights, the European Convention on Human Rights (www.hri.org/docs/ECHR50.html), informed the development of the UK Human Rights Act 1998 (www.opsi.gov.uk/acts/acts1998.htm), which has in turn brought about changes in health care practice, for example in seeking consent for treatment and care procedures (DOH 2001). The Convention also informed the Data Protection Act of 1998 (www.information commissioner.gov.uk), which has led health professionals to think more deeply about patient confidentiality.

Third is the nursing profession itself. The revised Code of Professional Conduct reflected the impact of the human rights legislation and the changes that had taken place in society during the preceding decade (Nursing and Midwifery Council (NMC) 2002; www.nmc-uk.org). The Code provides guidance about the standards of care that nurses should provide. Failure to comply with those standards can lead to a practitioner appearing before the Professional Conduct Committee.

Over to you

Look up the websites listed here and make brief notes about each document.

1. European Charter of Fundamental Rights and Freedoms (www.europarl.eu.int/charter)

2. European Convention on Human Rights (www.hri.org/docs/ECHR50.html)

3. Human Rights Act 1998 (www.opsi.gov.uk/acts/acts1998.htm); scroll down to Human Rights Act 1998

4. Data Protection Act 1998 (www.opsi.gov.uk/acts/acts1998.htm); scroll down to Data Protection Act 1998

Finally, there are policy influences. The UK general election of 1997 was followed by significant reforms of the National Health Service. These reforms were intended to modernise various aspects of service delivery, improve access to services and raise standards (DOH 1997; NHSE 1999; DOH 2000). The ways in which politicians conceptualise nursing have implications for the provision of care and have been instrumental in expanding care roles because nursing is currently regarded as being ideally placed to enable health services to meet the aims of the reforms.

In considering these factors, we can see that care cannot be considered in isolation from the rest of society. Care as a focus for nursing is not a matter solely for the profession but one that is subject to a number of external influences. In the end, nurses have to address how best to provide the care that society needs and wants to an acceptable professional standard for which the political frameworks provide funding.

Key points Top tips

- The provision of care is influenced by society's needs and expectations.
- Patients have greater access to information and therefore may need more help in making informed decisions.
- The Human Rights documents have influenced both UK law and professional thinking about care.

Conclusion

This chapter has helped you to begin to examine critically the concept of care in nursing by introducing a wide range of ideas. In doing so, it has become clear that care is not a single entity but a multifaceted concept that is influenced by our experiences as human beings. The study of care urges us to think about how we value people other than ourselves and the value they place on us. Care is a reciprocal activity based on giving and receiving, and in placing care at the centre of nursing we raise questions about what it is that patients can expect from us and what they might give us in return. Subsequent chapters in this book will help you to examine these questions further.

References

Adams, D. (2002) *The Salmon of Doubt*. London, Balantine Press.

Benner, P. and Wrubel, J. (1989) *The Primacy of Caring. Stress and Coping in Health and Illness*. Menlo Park CA, Addison Wesley Publishing Company.

Brechin, A. (2000) 'Introducing critical practice', Chapter 2 in A. Brechin, H. Brown and M. Eby (eds) *Critical Practice in Health and Social Care*. Buckingham, Open University Press, pp. 25–47.

De Bono, E. (2004) *Six Thinking Hats*. London, Penguin.

Department of Health (DOH) (1997) *The New NHS. Modern, Dependable*. London, DOH.

Department of Health (DOH) (1999) *Making a Difference: Strengthening the Nursing, Midwifery and Health Visiting Contribution to Health and Healthcare*. London, DOH.

Department of Health (DOH) (2000) *The NHS Plan. A Plan for Investment. A Plan for Reform*. London, DOH.

Department of Health (DOH) (2001) *Reference Guide to Consent for Examination or Treatment*. London, DOH, March.

Department of Health (DOH) (2003) *Choice, Responsiveness and Equity in the NHS and Social Care. A National Consultation*, London, DOH.

Eby, M. (2000) 'Understanding professional development', Chapter 3 in A. Brechin, H. Brown and M. Eby (eds) *Critical Practice in Health and Social Care*. Buckingham, Open University Press, pp. 48–70.

Edwards, S. D. (2001) *Philosophy of Nursing. An Introduction*. Houndmills, Basingstoke, Palgrave.

Hardey, M. (2001) 'Doctor in the house: the Internet as a source of lay knowledge and the challenge to expertise', Chapter 68 in B. Davey, A. Gray and C. Seale (eds) *Health and Disease: A Reader*. Buckingham, Open University Press, pp. 400–5.

Kleinman, A. (1988) *The Illness Narratives*. New York, Basic Books.

Leininger, M. (1984) *Care: the Essence of Nursing and Healthcare*. Detroit MI, Wayne State University Press.

Leininger, M. and McFarland, M. (2002) *Transcultural Nursing: Concepts, Theories, Research and Practice*, 3rd edn. New York, McGraw Hill.

McGee, P. (2000) *Culturally-sensitive Nursing: A Critique*. Unpublished PhD thesis, Birmingham, University of Central England.

National Health Service Executive (NHSE) (1999) *Nurse, Midwife and Health Visitor Consultants Health Service Circular* 1999/217.

Needleman, J., Beurhaus, P., Mattke, S., Stewart, M. and Zelebinsky, K. (2002) 'Nurse staffing levels and the quality of care in hospitals', *New England Journal of Medicine* 346 (22) pp. 1715–22.

Nursing and Midwifery Council (NMC) (2002) *Code of Professional Conduct*. London, NMC.

Oberle, K. and Allen, M. (2001) 'The nature of advanced nursing practice', *Nursing Outlook* 49 (3) pp. 148–53.

Royal College of Nursing (RCN) (2000) *Defining Nursing*. London, RCN.

Smith, P. (1992) *The Emotional Labour of Nursing*. London, Macmillan.

Watson, J. (1999) *Nursing, Human Science and Human Care. A Theory of Nursing*. Boston MA, Jones and Bartlett Publishers and National League for Nursing.

2

Receiving care

Learning outcomes

By the end of this chapter you should be able to:

- briefly explain the focus of nursing knowledge and the function of nursing as a service to society;

- apply your critical skills in examining the different patient groups for whom you provide care;

- relate your new knowledge to patients' experiences of good quality care;

- begin to understand some of the issues surrounding lack of care.

Introduction

Professional nursing care is intentionally directed towards others, either individually or as members of groups such as families, communities or places of work. The aims of that care are:

> to assist the individual, sick or well, in the performance of those activities contributing to health or its recovery (or to a peaceful death) that he would perform unaided if he had the necessary strength, will or knowledge. And to do this in such a way as to help him gain independence as rapidly as possible.
>
> (Henderson 1966 p. 15)

Care is thus relational, requiring intellectual and practical effort to achieve these aims, and creativity in meeting the needs of both the sick and dying as well as preventing illness or improving health.

Over to you

Look up two other definitions of nursing and compare and contrast these with each other and also with what Henderson has said. Which do you think most closely reflects the realities of nursing practice in your field? Give reasons for your argument.

Care requires an extensive and sophisticated knowledge base that in nursing is focused around four key elements (Fawcett 2000) – see Figure 2.1. The *person* is the recipient of care as an individual or as a member of a group. The *environment* refers to the settings in which care may take place and may include the physical environments of home, school, the wider community or hospital as well as the psychological environment of the individual or the social environment in which that person lives. *Health* refers to the person's state of being, i.e. what is normal for that individual.

●━ᵣ *Keywords*

Metaparadigm
A statement that defines the focus of a profession, outlining the main areas with which it is concerned and establishing boundaries between that profession and other activities.

Focusing on health rather than illness enables nurses to adopt a holistic approach to those for whom they provide care by contextualising those individuals' health problems or illnesses within their daily lives. Finally, *nursing* refers to the systematic undertaking of assessment, planning, implementation and evaluation. These four elements are referred to as the **metaparadigm** of nursing, that is, a series of statements that identify what nursing is and the functions it performs. If nursing has a body of knowledge centred on the person, health, the environment and nursing, then it incorporates an understanding of human beings in relation to their life processes and optimal functioning, behaviour and interaction with the environment in both normal life events and during illness. Nursing provides holistic services and interventions that contribute towards improvements in health (Fawcett 2000). This chapter begins with an examination of the metaparadigm and then helps you to examine the concept of the person in more detail, with particular reference to the experience of receiving nursing care.

> ## Over to you
>
> Read Carper, B. (1978) 'Fundamental patterns of knowing in nursing', *Advances in Nursing Science* 1 (1) pp. 13–23:
> 1 What does Carper say about the nature of nursing?
> 2 Compare and contrast her ideas with Fawcett's metaparadigm?
> 3 Which of the two is closest in your view to nursing in your field?

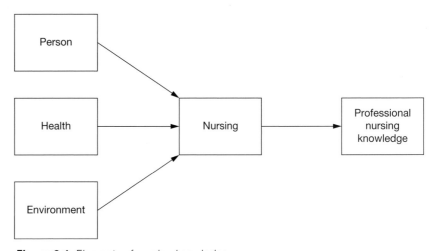

Figure 2.1 *Elements of nursing knowledge*

The metaparadigm of nursing

In critically appraising the extent to which the metaparadigm actually reflects modern nursing knowledge and practice it is useful to examine each of the four parts separately.

To begin with the concept of the *person*, which is simply a term for a human being, we can see that nursing activities are directed towards caring for human beings irrespective of any characteristics they may possess. Nurse theorists view the person as someone who is self-aware, conscious and able to think and to make decisions (Locke 1976). This view helps nurses to see that individual holistically, as having physical, psychological, social and spiritual dimensions, and as capable of taking an active role in their care. However, there is no single agreed view of what constitutes a person, so a lot hinges on the meanings that the profession attaches to this term. Nurse theorists have criticised mechanistic arguments based on the idea that mind and body are separate and that the body is no more than an interrelating set of physiological systems. System disease or breakdown requires a specific focus and treatment. Nurse theorists argue that the person is an intelligent being who is able to take an active part in maintaining health or managing illness. However, many patients are unable to do either, and this raises the possibility that they may not be regarded as persons (Allmark 1994).

The *environment* reflects the multiplicity of settings in which nursing care can take place. Nursing care in one environment may be quite different to that in another. Focusing on the environment also helps nurses to appreciate the relationship between the environment and health and the extent to which individuals or groups may be able to improve their health by altering the setting in which they live or work. The importance of the environment is particularly evident in Nightingale's (1860/1969) theory in terms of the impact this may have on health. Subsequent theorists have explored this impact from different perspectives. However, the environment in nursing theories is not consistently defined and is frequently the least well-developed aspect of individual theorists' work (see for example the work of Roper *et al.* 2000, Roy and Andrews 1999 and Travelbee 1971). Moreover, none of these theories addresses the relationship between the nurse and the environment and the ways in which this may impact on care.

The focus on *health* broadens the scope of nursing, moving it away from concentrating only on illness. This facilitates nursing care that promotes health through, for example, education, immunisation and other activities. However, health is a vague concept. It can be seen as a commodity that can be bought, for example, through care packages or private health insurance (Benner and Wrubel 1989).

Alternatively it can be viewed as an ideal state (World Health Organization (WHO) 1946). While the focus on health enables nurses to see that there is more to consider than the presence or absence of illness, it may also serve to make the boundaries of nursing vague and apparently limitless (Seedhouse 1998).

Finally, *nursing* unites the other three elements to ensure a holistic approach based on the recognition that individuals are in constant interaction with the environment and that this in turn affects their health. The focus on nursing challenges the profession to be explicit about what it offers to society and the ways in which this may vary. On the other hand, this focus is, according to Leininger (1984), somewhat tautological in that nursing is a phenomenon that requires clear explanation, and using the term nursing as one of the four elements of professional knowledge does not help to clarify nursing activities. In addition, the focus on nursing ignores the nurse as the provider of care, the ways in which individual characteristics may affect care delivery and the effects of caring on care givers (Travelbee 1971; Benner and Wrubel 1989; Smith 1992). (For more information on this subject see the sources listed in the 'Further reading' section at the end of this chapter.)

The person as a recipient of nursing care

As we have seen in the debate about the elements of nursing knowledge, the person can be regarded in several different ways. Nursing constantly emphasises that each individual is unique while at the same time adopting uniform approaches to care that ignore and suppress that individuality.

Reflective activity

Someone asks you where you are working at the moment. How do you respond? How do you describe the people for whom you provide care?

In the reflective activity you may have said 'I work in an orthopaedic ward' or 'I work as a district nurse', but this does not convey either the complexity of patients' needs or their levels of dependency. We need to look again at our patients and think about the different groups for whom we are providing care. For example, in an orthopaedic ward we are likely to encounter older people with chronic conditions such as osteoarthritis who are undergoing joint replacement, younger people with sporting injuries, those with deformities such as kyphosis and others with malignant disease (see Figures 2.2 and 2.3). Each of these patient groups requires particular approaches to care based on differing levels of dependency. For some, the hospital ward will be almost a home from home as they need lengthy or frequent periods of admission. Others will be admitted only once – for surgery such as joint replacement that will transform their mobility and quality of life. All are likely to experience pain and reduced or impaired mobility at some point, and for some there is the risk of permanent disability.

Reflective activity

Who are we providing care for?

Take a sheet of paper and think again about the patients for whom you provide care. Using Figures 2.2 and 2.3 as guides, identify the different patient groups. In what ways do the patients in each group rely on nursing care? In what ways are they independent of nursing care?

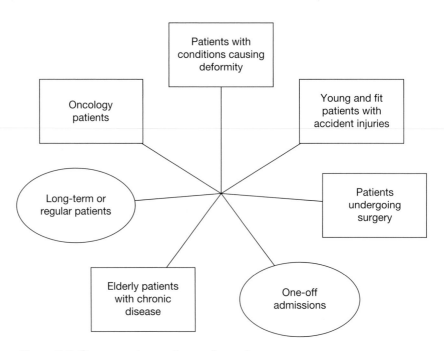

Figure 2.2 *The person in an orthopaedic ward*

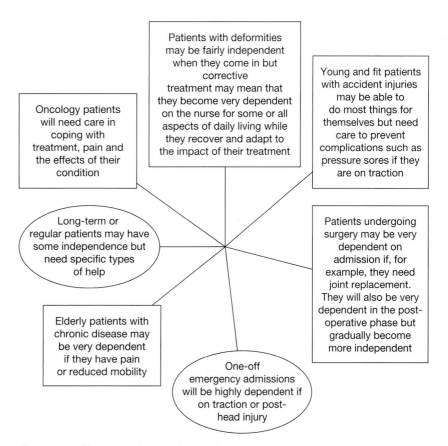

Figure 2.3 *The person in an orthopaedic ward – dependence versus independence*

This second exercise helps to make explicit the ways in which patient groups differ in terms of both their conditions and the degree of nursing interventions required. Imposing single approaches to care negates the differences between patient groups, a situation in which the provision of care is reduced to a 'one size fits all' approach. Furthermore, thinking about our particular patient groups helps to ensure that we see them more clearly as people like ourselves and leads us into considering how they may experience the care we provide.

Key points Top tips

- The metaparadigm of nursing clarifies the role and functions of nursing in society.
- The metaparadigm has four elements: person, health, environment and nursing.
- Each theory of nursing provides a particular interpretation of the four elements of the metaparadigm.
- The person is the recipient of nursing care, i.e. the patient.
- Patients' needs and levels of dependency will vary according to the underlying nature of their health problems and their individual circumstances.
- Individualised approaches to care are essential if nurses are to meet patients' needs and dependency.

Patients' experience of nursing care

Considering how patients might experience care is a challenge for those who give it to them. Just as we cannot experience the suffering of others, so we cannot know what it is to be on the receiving end of our care-giving activities. We can rely only on how people react to our interventions, what they tell us about these reactions and what we ourselves have learned as recipients of care from others.

Reflective activity

Being cared for

Identify one experience in which you felt that another person cared for or about you. Which aspects of that experience led you to feel cared for?

Identify one experience in which you felt that someone was uncaring towards you? Which aspects of that experience did you feel were uncaring?

Make a list of caring and uncaring attributes from these two experiences.

Patients' experiences of good quality care

Reflecting about our own experiences of receiving care can help us to understand how patients may interpret ideas about our nursing activities. McGee (2000) interviewed fifty-four patients who had recently been discharged from acute hospital wards in four different

National Health Service (NHS) Trusts about their experiences. The outcomes revealed four categories of activities that patients perceived as good care given to them by nurses:

1   care as an interpersonal skill;

2   care as showing concern;

3   care as practical help;

4   care as performance.

Care as an interpersonal skill

The term **interpersonal skill** refers to a range of activities and behaviours through which we interact with other people. Successful interaction depends on our ability to pay attention to others, listen to what they say and respond with verbal and non-verbal messages that are meaningful to them. Inherent in the exercise of interpersonal skills are factors such as personality, attitudes and beliefs. Nursing requires highly developed interpersonal skills based on an understanding and awareness of the self and reflection about how others may react to the self. Technical proficiency and clinical expertise are not enough. To provide effective care the nurse must also be able to communicate effectively and develop an understanding of the patient's perspective of the situation (Spross *et al.* 2000).

McGee (2000) found that the application of interpersonal skills in the provision of care began with the ward environment created by the nurses. The best wards had a family atmosphere in which nurses addressed patients by their first names. Patients valued the manner in which nurses spoke them. This was not just about politeness. Patients felt that they were special people, simply because of the way in which the nurses spoke to them. Nurses who came straightaway when called, who were not impatient and did not keep people waiting helped to enhance this feeling of being special. Feeling special created a basis for interactions that were more intimate or individualised. Patients welcomed nurses who explained everything before they did it and taught people how to perform tasks such as putting on anti-embolism stockings, rather than just leaving them to struggle. Competence in interpersonal skills, therefore, seems to have been experienced at two levels, the private and personal as well as the more public environment of the ward as a whole.

⊶ Keywords

Interpersonal skill

A range of activities and behaviours through which we interact with other people.

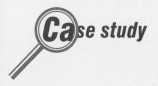

Case study

Mr Taylor has to ask the nurse for a urine bottle for the third time. He apologises to the nurse: 'I know you're very busy. I'm sorry to be a trouble to you.'

How often do we keep patients waiting, saying, 'I'll be there in a minute', or even forget altogether that they have asked for something? Why do you think Mr Taylor thinks he has to apologise?

Care as showing concern

McGee found that nurses demonstrated concern for patients by asking them how they were and offering cups of tea 'so that you were made to feel that they were paying attention to you' (Patient 1). This was considered particularly important as patients recovered from illness or surgery and especially when their beds were moved down the ward, away from the nurses' station. The layout of some wards could leave patients feeling that they rarely saw a nurse. Someone who came round to each bed and asked how each person was feeling was therefore welcomed as a form of reassurance. Patients spoke warmly about members of staff who recognised when people were feeling distressed and who stopped and listened, tried to help or perhaps gave someone a hug when nothing else could be done (McGee 2000).

Reflective activity

To what extent do you:

- make time, in every shift, to check on patients who are designated as self-caring?
- genuinely not have time to check on them as often as you would like?
- neglect patients who no longer require physical care?

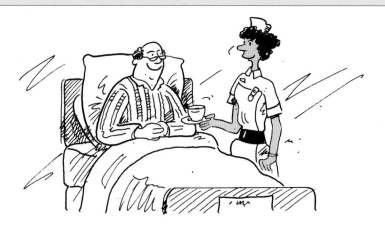

Care as practical help

McGee found that patients valued practical help that enabled them to cope with specific problems such as managing incontinence, getting out of bed on the first day after an operation or performing everyday activities such as taking a bath. Practical help was important because it helped patients to achieve what they had previously thought impossible and also created opportunities to talk about worries and fears. Nurses who listened to patients' concerns and who tried to help, made suggestions or provided telephone contacts to be followed up later were considered particularly caring. Receiving practical help was important but it was the interpersonal competence of the nurse that transformed it into care, indicating that the nature of care lies not just in what is done but in the manner in which actions are performed (McGee 2000).

Care as performance

McGee found that the quality of nurses' actions changed the nature of even routine activities, suggesting that certain aspects of care are embedded in performance (McGee 2000). Such skills can be demonstrated but are difficult to describe or teach formally.

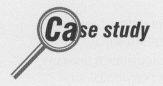

Case study

Read the two case studies below.

Bertha Jones was an elderly woman who had been in hospital for several weeks following surgery:

> I was now able to do most things for myself and was hoping to go home in a few days. Normally I have to get up once during the night to go to the toilet but this one particular night I had to get up several times. No sooner had I got back into bed than I would have to get up again and on one trip to the toilet I wet the floor. Oh, I was so embarrassed and didn't tell anyone. It went on all the next day. I was that worried about wetting the bed during the night. Nurse Jackson, the night nurse, the second night, she saw me making trips to the toilet and asked if I was alright. I didn't know what to say to her but she seemed to just know already what the problem was. When I came out of the toilet one time, she took me aside and seemed to know what questions to ask. You know, 'Does it sting when you have to pass water? Are you finding you have to go far more often?' She said she thought that I had an infection in my water and that I needed some antibiotics. I didn't tell her about wetting myself but she seemed to know that this could happen so I didn't have to bring it up. She said 'You're not to worry if you can't get to the toilet in time. It often happens with this sort of infection. If it happens just tell me. I'm here to help you with this sort of thing. And I don't want you to slip on a wet floor. Next time you go to the toilet I will take a sample of your urine and get it tested.' And she did and she got me started on these tablets. A day or so later I was fine. And she moved the bed into a side ward where it had like an en suite so I didn't have so far to go.

Jo Mercer, a middle-aged woman, was recovering from a hysterectomy:

> Every morning, the physiotherapist came to the ward to teach these pelvic floor exercises. She had a class in the day room, and we were all supposed to go. She'd go round saying 'Come on girls. Girls she always called us. Mind you she was only a girl herself. Come on girls. We don't want to have continence problems when we get home, do we?' Well you can imagine. We went the first day and it was awful. Just didn't know what she was on about half the time. Kept thinking it must be lunchtime soon. There she was banging on about continence problems (whatever they were). And the way she talked it was like you were back at school. Anyway the next day no one wanted to be bothered but the nurses kind of got everybody rounded up, like you couldn't say no without upsetting them and then two of them, the nurses, they joined in with us. What a laugh! They kept cracking these jokes till we nearly wet ourselves. Then they'd ask questions and like make the physio explain things. And she said it was about making sure you didn't wet yourself. And we sort of got into sex, well it was all women, and well you could see the point. But we had such a laugh. And those nurses, they must have done it all a hundred times but it was like they were doing it for the first time, just like us. We had such a laugh. It was great!

What does each patient experience as caring?

Nursing skills can appear deceptively simple, especially when they are an integral part of an expert nurse's repertoire. In such circumstances the performance of even routine activities represents a way of being with patients that takes account of emotional and physical responses and the needs of each individual (McGee 2000; Benner *et al.* 1996). In other words, skills become embodied, a part of the practitioner concerned, and performance goes beyond initial expectations. Nurses can easily learn to deal with urinary tract infections or the conduct of pelvic floor exercises, but to do so day after day, in ways that make patients feel special or entertained, requires a high level of interpersonal skills matched with clinical and technical expertise that enables the practitioner to hone in accurately on a problem and what it means for the patient at an emotional level. In the examples presented in this chapter the nurses seemed to anticipate how the patient felt. The nurses were attuned to the situation, involved in ways that enabled them to respond with kindness as well as clinically sound decisions without allowing themselves to become overwhelmed. For them, caring involved learning 'safe and helpful closeness and distance' through interpersonal connections (Benner *et al.* 1999).

Key points Top tips

- Reflecting on your own experiences of being cared for will help you to understand what it feels like to receive care and how patients may feel about the care you provide.
- Care giving requires highly developed interpersonal skills that enable nurses to connect with patients, anticipating their difficulties and their feelings.
- Good interpersonal skills create care environments in which patients feel that they matter, that they are important.
- Patients value care environments in which nurses use their interpersonal skills to show concern for patients.
- Care has practical, clinical and technical as well as interpersonal dimensions.
- Skilled nurses synthesise interpersonal skills with professional knowledge and skills to identify accurately patients' problems and meet their individual needs.

Patients' experiences of lack of care

McGee's study showed that patients' experiences of lack of care were associated with what is often referred to as *basic nursing*, that is to say those activities identified as fundamental to individual well-being but taken for granted until sickness, or disability, renders them problematic. Washing oneself, performing mouth care, eating, drinking, moving around and breathing easily are essential in providing comfort and creating a situation in which more sophisticated interventions can be used to good effect (Roper *et al.* 2000). Poor hydration and inappropriate positioning will negate the effects of administering antibiotics for a chest infection. Lack of attention to mouth care may lead to the development of further infection and possible gum disease. Lack of attention to mobility may result in bedsores. All of these possibilities are avoidable through the application of basic nursing. Nurses need to recognise the value of basic nursing and retain it as a central part of their work alongside the new technical and clinical skills required in health care.

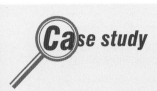

Case study

Albert Staines was an elderly man who had been admitted to hospital with a severe chest infection:

The morning after they took me in I felt bad, really bad. I'd no strength in me. I was just lying there like a baby. Couldn't move myself. Couldn't get out of bed. Couldn't do nothing. And during the night I must have been sweating like because the sheets felt damp. I thought, 'I must smell.' Well no one came to give you a wash. They brought the breakfast round and they put this tray on the table at the end of the bed but I couldn't reach it and my mouth it felt like there was fur growing in it. Anyway someone else came and took it [the tray] away. Mind you I didn't want anything. A bit later on one of the other chaps he comes up to me and he says, 'How are you?' I said, 'Oh, could you get me a glass of water, anything to drink.' Anyway he brought me this glass of water and I drank it straight off. Down in one. And the rest of the day that's what he did. He kept bringing me water, and cups of tea because, he said, there was a machine for patients in the day room wherever that was. They brought round the dinner and the tea but I couldn't reach and I, well, I didn't like to ask him to do too much. In case he took offence you know. They brought the tablets round. Otherwise you were on your own.

The next morning I felt just as bad and this nurse I'd never seen before she comes up and says 'How are you feeling?' I said, 'I feel rough and I could do with a wash. I never had one yesterday.' And straight away she gets this chair on wheels and she wheels me to the shower. She was so good. She showered me down, which was wonderful. And when she took me back to the bed, and it was all fresh like, she gave me this bell and she said, 'Now you ring me when you want anything.' She was good she was. On the job.

What does the patient experience as a lack of caring?

Whether or not patients receive good quality care seems to be a matter of individual responses to a situation. In the case study above it is possible that no one intended harm towards Albert Staines; there was no conscious decision to deliberately neglect him, but nevertheless that is what happened. If questioned, the nurses working on the ward might have argued that they were short of staff, that an agency nurse was allocated to that part of the ward, that each thought the other had attended to this patient, that the medicine round took longer than anticipated. All sorts of excuses could be put forward as reasons for what happened, but if nurses were not responsible, then who was? Nurses, and only nurses, are trained and employed to ensure that people such as Albert Staines receive help with those activities that they cannot perform for themselves. It is their proper role. While hospital wards are very busy and there is a limit to what each member of staff can accomplish in any shift, nurses excuse neglect by arguing that there is not time to do even the essentials. Once in a while this may be so, but nurses, and other health professionals, hide behind this argument too often and too easily. Rather than there being a genuine lack of time, it is possible that some practitioners really cannot be bothered, that care may not be the universal phenomenon that Leininger (1984) claims it to be. Nevertheless, patients try to meet nurses half way, absolving the lack of care and other shortcomings, preferring to regard nurses as overworked with too many people to care for and no time to make friends with patients or treat them as individuals. Members of staff are under great pressure, resulting in lapses in care rather than deliberate non-caring. Thus nurses and patients construct their own explanations of lack of care in ways that save face for both parties. Patients are dependent on nurses not only for their care but also for other aspects of their stay in hospital. Neither they nor the nurses see it as being in their interests to confront neglect openly. Fudging the issue allows both sides to maintain the business of running the ward (McGee 2000).

Key points | Top tips

- Patients experience a lack of care when nurses do not help them with the activities of living that they are unable to perform for themselves.
- Lack of care may cause patients to experience further, preventable complications.
- Lack of care may result when nurses are genuinely overworked.
- Patients make excuses when care is not forthcoming in order to avoid difficulties in their dealings with nurses.
- Nurses have to confront their own shortcomings over the provision of care and not hide behind excuses when care has been omitted.

Conclusion

This chapter has helped you to apply a critical approach to the examination of nursing as a service provided to society. That service centres around the four key elements of person, health, environment and nursing and facilitates an understanding of both health and illness and the provision of care that addresses individual needs. In considering such needs you have started to identify the different groups of persons for whom you provide care and the ways in which they may experience your interventions. The next chapter enables you to look at care giving from your perspective as a nurse and to determine the extent to which your intentions and experiences may match with those of patients.

Rapid recap

1   Why should nurses adopt a different nursing approach according to the needs of each patient group?

2   How can we consider how patients might experience the care given to them?

3   What four aspects of care do patients perceive as indicators of good care from nurses?

4   What aspect of nursing care do patients most commonly find is lacking?

References

Allmark, P. (1994) 'An argument against the use of the concept of "persons" in health care ethics', *Journal of Advanced Nursing* 19 pp. 29–35.

Benner, P. and Wrubel, J. (1989) *The Primacy of Caring. Stress and Coping in Health and Illness.* Menlo Park CA, Addison Wesley Publishing Company.

Benner, P., Tanner, C. and Chesla, C. (1996) *Expertise in Nursing Practice. Caring, Clinical Judgement and Ethics.* New York, Springer Publishing Company.

Benner, P., Hooper-Kyriakidis, P. and Stannard, D. (1999) *Clinical Wisdom and Interventions in Critical Care: A Thinking-in-action Approach.* Philadelphia PA, W. B. Saunders.

Carper, B. (1978) 'Fundamental patterns of knowing in nursing', *Advances in Nursing Science* 1 (1) pp. 13–23.

Fawcett, J. (2000) *Analysis and Evaluation of Contemporary Nursing Knowledge: Nursing Models and Theories*, 2nd edn. Philadelphia PA, F. A. Davis.

Henderson, V. (1966) *The Nature of Nursing*. New York, Macmillan.

Leininger, M. (1984) *Care: the Essence of Nursing and Healthcare*. Detroit MI, Wayne State University Press

Locke, J. (1976) *An Essay Concerning Human Understanding*. Oxford, Oxford University Press.

McGee, P. (2000) *Culturally-sensitive Nursing: A Critique*. Unpublished PhD thesis, Birmingham, University of Central England.

Nightingale, N. (1860/1969) *Notes on Nursing: What It Is and What It Is Not.* New York, Dover Publications.

Roper, N., Logan, W. and Tierney, A. (2000) *The Roper-Logan-Tierney Model of Nursing: Based on Activities of Living*. Edinburgh, Churchill Livingstone.

Roy, C. and Andrews, H. (1999) *The Roy Adaptation Model*. Stamford CT, Appleton and Lange.

Seedhouse, D. (1998) *Ethics: the Heart of Health Care*, 2nd edn. Chichester, John Wiley and Son.

Smith, P. (1992) *The Emotional Labour of Nursing*. London, Macmillan.

Spross, J., Clarke, E. and Baggerley, J. (2000) 'Expert coaching and guidance', Chapter 7 in A. Hamric, J. Spross and C. Hanson (eds) *Advanced Nursing Practice. An Integrative Approach*, 2nd edn. Philadelphia PA, W. B. Saunders, pp. 183–216.

Travelbee, J. (1971) *Interpersonal Aspects of Nursing*. Philadelphia PA, F. A. Davis.

World Health Organization (WHO) (1946) *Constitution*. Geneva, WHO.

Further reading

Benner, P. (1984) *Novice to Expert: Excellence and Power in Clinical Nursing Practice,* Menlo Park CA, Addison Wesley.

Levine, M. (1967) 'The four conservation principles of nursing', *Nursing Forum* 6 p. 45.

Neuman's systems theory in: Neuman, B. and Fawcett, J. (2002) *The Neuman Systems Model*. Upper Saddle River NJ, Prentice Hall.

Nightingale's theory in: Nightingale, N. (1860/1969) *Notes on Nursing: What It Is and What It Is Not*. New York, Dover Publications.

Orem's theory of self-care in: Orem, D. (2001) *Nursing, Concepts of Practice*, 6th edn. St Louis MO, C. V. Mosby.

Roy's theory of adaptation in: Roy, C. and Andrews, H. (1999) *The Roy Adaptation Model*. Stamford CT, Appleton and Lange.

Readers unable to obtain copies of any of these texts will find the following text helpful:

Marriner Tomey, A. and Alligood, M. R. (2002) (eds) *Nursing Theorists and Their Work*, 5th edn. St Louis MO, Mosby.

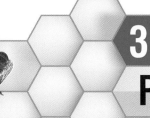

3

Providing care

Learning outcomes

By the end of this chapter you should be able to:

- critically appraise theoretical ideas about nursing;
- apply your critical skills to an examination of different approaches to the assessment of your patients;
- understand the concept of nursing diagnosis and begin to formulate nursing diagnoses for your patients;
- apply your new knowledge to planning care for patients.

Introduction

According to Fawcett (2000), contemporary nursing knowledge is expressed in a metaparadigm consisting of four elements. These elements are neutral, that is to say that there is no single way in which they should be viewed or interpreted. Instead, they provide the basis for individual members of the profession to formulate philosophies and theories that inform both nurses and non-nurses about the nature of nursing. Each theory presents a particular view of what nursing is, depending on the author's background, interests and field of practice. There is not, and indeed cannot be, a single theory to which everyone must subscribe, because nursing is so diverse, serving so many different groups of people in a wide variety of settings. The lack of a single theory for nursing facilitates intellectual debate and the incorporation of new ideas as practice changes.

Over to you

Comparing and contrasting theoretical ideas about nursing

Select one nursing theory text, for example Marriner Tomey, A. and Alligood, M. R. (eds) (2002) *Nursing Theorists and Their Work*, 5th edn. St Louis MO, Mosby. Choose any two chapters about individual theories of nursing and summarise information about the background of the two theorists, for example their fields of practice, the period in which they wrote, the influences to which they were exposed etc., and what each has to say about the nature of the person, health, nursing and the environment.

Compare and contrast each summary.

How useful would each theory be in your own field of practice?

Thus individual practitioners have the opportunity to contribute to professional discourse by developing their own theoretical ideas. However, few have done so explicitly, especially outside the United States, and consequently there are not many published theories about the nature of nursing in the UK. Those that are available have been adopted as part of whole organisational approaches to nursing care that have tended to stifle new ideas and discouraged nurses from developing their own theories. From a managerial perspective, adopting a single theoretical approach to care can help to clarify the nature of nursing services to the Trust board and, in practice settings, ensure that all staff share the same frame of reference. This has repercussions for both theory and practice in attempting to match the two. Either the theory must somehow be made to fit with every possible care setting, including those for which it was not, in the first instance, intended or care is made to fit into a theoretical framework which is not really suited to the patient group concerned. This chapter helps you to examine the suitability of nursing theories for your practice with particular reference to assessing and planning care.

Theoretical approaches to nursing care

Professional nursing care takes place within a cyclical framework of assessment, planning, implementation and evaluation known as the *nursing process*. Assessment is conducted using a mixture of observation, measurement and **semi-structured interviewing** to obtain information about the physiological, social and psychological situation of the patient. The object of assessment is to focus on the patient as a unique individual and to utilise the information obtained to provide care that meets that person's situation. Assessment is performed when patients first come into contact with nursing services but may also take place as part of the appraisal of an individual's progress or to facilitate detailed exploration of a specific problem. Successful completion of an assessment is dependent on several factors. First, the nurse must possess interpersonal skills that can be used to constructively explore the patient's problems and build the foundations of a subsequent therapeutic relationship. Second, the patient must be willing to engage in the assessment by contributing information and by working with the nurse. Third, the nurse requires an assessment framework that guides the gathering and interpretation of information in ways that facilitate the formulation of accurate diagnoses. Assessment frameworks arise from nursing theories. Each theory provides a particular view of nursing and, as a part of this, ideas about how assessment should be carried out.

---

o─┬ *Keywords*

Semi-structured interviews

Those in which the interviewer asks questions based on a list of topics. The questions and topics can be covered in any order depending on how the conversation develops. Semi-structured interviews allow the nurse to explore topics of concern to the patient and gain a deep understanding of how that person experiences their particular health problems.

Structured interviews

Those in which the interviewer has a carefully prepared list of questions, similar to a questionnaire, and asks each in turn without any deviation in order or phrasing so that the questions asked are exactly the same in each interview. Market research interviews are one example of this type of interview.

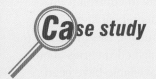

Sydney Green is a retired railway porter who lives alone following his divorce ten years ago. His main interests are horse racing and gardening in his allotment where he grows vegetables that he sells locally to augment his pension. He smokes two packets of cigarettes a day and has mild hypertension. During the last year he has experienced difficulties in passing urine and has to get up several times each night. He tends to pass small amounts and frequently experiences difficulties in starting the flow of urine. He has twice been admitted to hospital with acute retention of urine. Investigations have shown that his prostate gland is enlarged but he has refused surgery. However, after discussing it with his new partner, he has changed his mind and has come into hospital for a prostatectomy.

Using Roper *et al.*'s (2000) theory of nursing, show how you would assess this patient.

Repeat the exercise using another theory of nursing.

Compare and contrast the two assessments.

The work of Roper, Logan and Tierney has provided the most frequently used nursing theory for nursing practice in the UK (Roper *et al.* 2000). The theory promotes a holistic approach to patient care based on five elements that form the basis of assessment (see Figure 3.1). First, there is the notion of *individuality in living*, that no two people are exactly alike either as people or in the way in which they live their lives. Second, there are the *activities of living* that all individuals perform in a unique way and that may be affected by a change in health status that may arise because of the third element, namely *biological, psychological, sociocultural, politico-economic* or *environmental factors*. Fourth, each activity has to be considered in relation to the individual's *age* and *stage of development*. Finally, the person's *level of independence* or *dependence* must be taken into account with regard to each activity. Application of these ideas creates a two-tier assessment. The first part clarifies the individual's usual way of life and state of health, which in Sydney Green's case will help to expand on his normally independent lifestyle and the relationship with his partner. It may also help to ascertain the degree of social support that might be available to him as he recovers from surgery. The second level of assessment identifies the changes brought about by illness and disease, such as, in this case, the effects of interrupted sleep or possible backache if the prostate gland is very enlarged. These two levels of assessment provide the basis for planning individualised care (Roper *et al.* 2000).

In contrast to Roper *et al.* (2000), Levine (1969) proposed a view of nursing based on holism and *conservation*, that is to say the

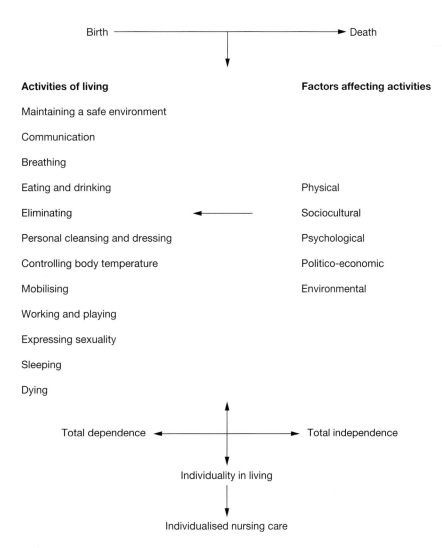

Figure 3.1 *Factors for assessment in Roper, Logan and Tierney's theory of nursing (based on Roper et al. 2000 pp. 14 and 78)*

Reflective activity

Nursing theory in your field of practice
What theory is currently used to underpin nursing practice in your workplace and why?

Is the theory used:

- completely, i.e. as the theorist intended?
- partially, i.e. selected parts of it are used?
- nominally, i.e. just the basic ideas?

To what extent is the use of this theory helpful in providing care?

individual's need to ensure physical and psychological integrity. The individual is composed of an internal environment of interrelated physical and psychological systems that are described as *homoeostatic*, that is energy sparing (Schaefer 2002). The internal environment is also *homeorhetic*, that is capable of adaptation to sustain well-being (Fawcett 2000). Individuals exist in a constant state of change within an external environment that they can perceive through their senses, that can affect them in ways that cannot be detected through the senses and that has a conceptual dimension based on language. Conservation refers to the individual's capacity to function and cope with change in ways that avoid the excessive use of energy while maintaining *structural* (physical), *personal* (identity and self-worth) and *social integrity* (Levine 1966a; Schaefer 2002). Health is defined by the individual and by the social groups to which that person belongs. Thus health has cultural, social, psychological and physiological dimensions. Health is maintained through the appropriate use of adaptive skills. For example, inflammation is an appropriate response that facilitates healing (Schaefer 2002). Illness results from anarchic patterns of adaptation. The goal of nursing is conservation, that is, to enable the patient to adapt positively to changes in health by working collaboratively with that person (Levine 1967).

Assessment of a patient using Levine's theory requires the nurse to focus on the conservation of energy by determining the extent to which that person can perform activities without fatigue (see Figure 3.2). This requires the nurse to consider the adaptive processes that the individual may have used and the extent to which these are appropriate. Assessment of conservation of structural integrity requires the collection of information about physiological processes including vital signs, physical functions and pain. In considering adaptation, Sydney Green may have tried to reduce his night-time visits to the toilet by reducing the amount of fluids he drinks, thus increasing the risk of urinary tract infection. Assessment of conservation of personal integrity requires an exploration of the individual's values and expectations; for example, self-esteem, desire and ability to participate in decision-making and expectations of professionals. In Sydney Green's case, this aspect of assessment might include his understanding of prostatectomy and the possible long-term physical effects that may impact on his new relationship. Assessment of conservation of social integrity includes identification of the patient's usual social networks and significant others. The assessment culminates in an interpretation of the information gained to ascertain the key factors in the patient's current health situation. These factors are used to inform a process that Levine called *trophicognosis*, the formulation of a nursing judgement (Levine 1966b; Fawcett 2000) that informs the planning and delivery of care (see Figure 3.2).

Both Roper *et al.* (2000) and Levine (1969) adopt a holistic view of patients and provide frameworks for assessment that enable the nurse to gather a wide range of information that is relevant to the care of a patient undergoing surgery. Roper *et al.* (2000) communicate their theory in simple, familiar and easy-to-understand terms that make it seem simple to apply. However, clarity and simplicity of expression should not be confused with the actual theoretical ideas, which are both wide-ranging and complex (Chinn and Kramer 2004). Levine's (1969) theory is much older than that of Roper *et al.* (2000) and is expressed in a different style. She uses terms like 'trophicognosis' that are unfamiliar and at times difficult to understand. While this can be helpful in provoking us to think carefully about her theoretical ideas, Levine (1969) also serves to exemplify one of the continuing challenges besetting theorists in nursing, namely the language that they use. Each discipline has a professional language that acts as a short cut for members to communicate information, but it also serves to exclude those who do not understand the terminology used. Nursing theory is a discipline, with a professional language, but beyond the metaparadigm there is little consistent terminology. The use of arcane language serves to alienate most practitioners and may even, at times, obscure inadequately developed ideas. It is hardly surprising that many nurses hold negative views about theory and accuse theorists of not living in the real world. There is no doubt that nursing theory has an image problem that would be greatly improved by communicating complex ideas in plain language that the majority of nurses find meaningful and helpful.

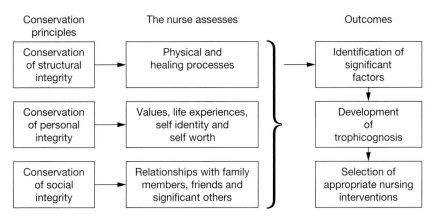

Figure 3.2 *Levine's theory of the conservation of energy*

Reflec**Reflective activity**

Think back to the first time you listened to nurses giving a verbal handover report. How much did you understand? Think about how you give handover reports now. Is information communicated as clearly as it could be? Are new, less experienced colleagues and students in any way disadvantaged by the use of specialist terminology? How could handover reporting be improved in your place of work?

Assessments using Roper *et al.*'s and Levine's theories provide broadly the same information, but there are some differences. For example, Levine's focus on personal integrity leads to a consideration of the patient's self-esteem – which, in the case of the patient in the case study above, may have been altered by his urinary problems. Personal integrity also raises the issue of the patient's beliefs. For example, the patient in the case study may think that the prostatectomy will affect his sexual function but feel unable to broach this subject. On the other hand, Roper *et al.*'s consideration of politico-economic factors may reveal concerns about his income while he is unable to earn extra from the sale of produce from his allotment. Thus each assessment has some unique and pertinent insights to offer.

The two nursing theories discussed in this chapter set out clear guidance for assessment. Peplau (1952), whose theory focuses on interpersonal relations, did not do this. In her view the nurse–patient relationship was the most important factor. In the assessment the two meet as strangers and must, through this encounter, forge the basis of a therapeutic relationship. This relationship develops gradually from a beginning in which each party affords the other mutual respect. Assessment is unstructured, in the manner of normal conversation. Thus the nurse does not approach assessment with a preconceived checklist of questions to ask.

Theory into Practice

What are the advantages and disadvantages of applying Peplau's approach to assessment in your field of practice?

What matters is finding the most appropriate approach to assessment to meet the needs of the patients for whom we care, based on critical analysis, critical action and critical reflexivity to clarify:

- our knowledge and understanding of the particular health needs of our patients;
- the type of information that best enables us to provide care;
- the degree to which a theory is oriented towards our patient groups;
- the ease with which we can apply the theoretical ideas;
- the likely benefits of introducing change.

Key points Top tips

- There is no universal theory of nursing that is suitable for every patient group or care setting.
- Each nursing theory represents the views of a practitioner.
- Each nurse can contribute to professional discourse by developing theoretical ideas.
- Nursing theories are applied through the nursing process, which provides a framework for the assessment, planning, implementation and evaluation of care.
- Assessment requires a synthesis of clinical and technical expertise alongside highly developed interpersonal skills.
- The end product of assessment is the identification of the patient's problems and the formulation of a nursing diagnosis.

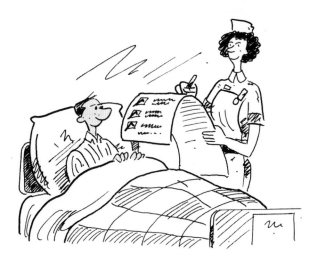

Nursing diagnosis

The end product of any nursing assessment is the identification of the patient's problems and the formulation of a *nursing diagnosis*. This is 'a clinical judgement about individual, family or community responses to actual or potential health problems/life processes. Nursing diagnosis provides the basis for selection of nursing interventions to achieve outcomes for which the nurse is responsible' (North American Nursing Diagnosis Association (NANDA) 1990). Thus a nursing diagnosis is a professional judgement, based on the nurse's understanding of the patient's situation, about factors that are within the sphere of nursing work and expressed in a way that is meaningful to other nurses and, where appropriate, to members of other disciplines. A nursing diagnosis forms the basis for planning care (Carpenito-Moyet 2004).

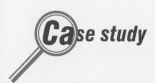

Case study

Mary MacGregor is 63 years old. She lives alone with her dog although her son and daughter live nearby. Mary usually looks after her son's and her daughter's children when they come home from school because both sets of parents work full time. On admission to hospital, nursing assessment shows that Mary has marked weakness in her right arm and leg creating difficulties with balance and movement. She has difficulties in feeding herself as well as chewing and swallowing her food. Her speech is difficult to understand because the right side of her face is also weak and saliva constantly dribbles from her mouth. She smokes 40 cigarettes a day and she has a chesty but ineffectual cough. She is slightly overweight and has been taking tablets to control her blood pressure.

Try to identify the nursing diagnoses you might make in this situation. Can you think of any difficulties that may arise in formulating these diagnoses? Use Roper *et al.*'s (2000) theory of nursing to help you.

The need to express nursing diagnoses clearly presents a challenge to practitioners. In assessing Mary MacGregor by using Roper *et al.*'s (2000) theory of nursing, you will have identified a number of problem areas that indicate a need for care. For example, she has a chesty, smoker's cough that you may have classified as a breathing problem or as a safety issue because of the risk of infection. Similarly, you may have described her impaired balance in terms of mobility or related it to her inability to feed herself. Thus one of the first issues in formulating nursing diagnoses is to ensure accuracy of expression. The technical language of medicine allows medical diagnoses to be formulated using terms that are understood clearly by everyone. In Mary MacGregor's case it is clear that she has a history of hypertension for which she is receiving medication. Doctors, nurses and other health professionals all share the same understanding of this term and are able to incorporate it into their own interventions. Until recently there has been no comparable technical language in nursing that allowed practitioners to convey their diagnoses in quite the same way. One attempt to address this

• Health promotion	• Sexuality
• Nutrition	• Coping/stress tolerance
• Elimination	• Life principles
• Activity/rest	• Safety/protection
• Perception/cognition	• Comfort
• Self-perception	• Growth/development
• Role relationships	

Figure 3.3 *Domains of nursing diagnoses*

situation can be seen in the work of the North American Nursing Diagnosis Association (NANDA) (www.nanda.org). Set up in 1982, the Association aims to develop and refine nursing diagnoses in thirteen domains (see Figure 3.3). Gradually the idea of nursing diagnosis has been exported to nursing in other countries and has recently been adopted by the International Council of Nurses (ICN) (www.icn.ch/icnpupdate.htm).

> ## Over to you
>
> Visit the NANDA website at www.nanda.org. What does this organisation do? What are the key publications produced by NANDA?
>
> Visit the ICN website at www.icn.ch. Click on ICNP® in the left-hand column, scroll down and click in ICNP® Beta 2 Version and then select 'guidelines for composing a nursing diagnosis'. Look back at one of the diagnoses that you identified for Mary MacGregor and re-state this in the light of the guidance provided on this website.

A second challenge in considering nursing diagnosis is the interface with medicine. While the work of NANDA has helped to clarify the distinct knowledge of nursing and the contribution it makes to patient care, the interface between nursing and medicine is constantly changing. The development of new, advanced roles in which activities that were previously in the medical domain have now become part of nursing practice has altered the historic patterns of interaction between the professions (Gidlow and Ellis 2003) causing some doctors to feel threatened by what they see as an erosion of their role (McGee 2003). In this context nursing diagnosis may be viewed as a source of potential conflict. However, it must be emphasised that nursing diagnoses are not intended to rival or supplant those of other professionals even though there may be occasions when medical and nursing judgements are very similar. Approaches to the development of advanced nursing roles in

Australia have shown that, by recruiting doctors to be active members of multidisciplinary working parties, nurses can not only facilitate the introduction of changes in their own practice but also enable medical practitioners to enthusiastically support such changes (Appel and Malcolm 1999).

A third challenge posed by nursing diagnosis is consideration of those issues that lie outside the domain of nursing. In Mary MacGregor's case there are two medical diagnoses, hypertension and cerebro-vascular accident, plus several other problems that will require the intervention of a speech therapist (to assess swallowing), a physiotherapist (to assess and improve movement and co-ordination), an occupational therapist (to assess and improve daily living skills) and others. The nurse will work closely with all these professions, as well as Mary's family, in caring for her and helping her to regain as much independence as possible. Working in this way takes the nurse outside the realm of nursing diagnosis towards *collaborative problems*, which may be monitored by the nurse but managed using a combination of interventions derived from nursing and other disciplines (Carpenito-Moyet 2004). Thus not all Mary MacGregor's problems are within the domain of nursing, but the nurse is responsible for identifying areas of need and ensuring that appropriate sources of help are secured.

Over to you

Read 'Nursing diagnoses: issues and controversies' in Carpenito-Moyet, L. J. (2004), pp. 68–75.

What additional issues in nursing diagnosis does the author explore?

Key points   Top tips

- A nursing diagnosis is a professional judgement, based on the nurse's understanding of the patient's situation, about factors that are within the sphere of nursing work and expressed in a way that is meaningful to other nurses.
- Nursing diagnoses are still developing because until recently there was no agreed terminology in which they might be expressed.
- NANDA and the ICN have helped to establish a definition of nursing diagnosis and guidelines for expressing diagnoses in practice.
- A nursing diagnosis does not rival or supplant a medical diagnosis.
- Some nursing diagnoses may indicate a need to involve members of other disciplines in patient care.
- Nursing diagnoses form the basis of care planning.

Planning and evaluating care

Providing care for patients requires the nurse to use the data gathered in assessment to establish priorities. Most nursing theories require that this be done in partnership with the patient although there may be occasions in which the individual's condition renders this impossible. *Partnership* with patients is an important principle, helping the nurse to maintain a focus on individualised care and to provide care that the patient both needs and wants. The notion of partnership also represents a move away from *compliance*, the traditional professional expectations that patients will simply do as they are told, and replaces this with the concept of *concordance*, that is to say, a negotiated plan that suits the individual's wishes and circumstances.

Reflective activity

Is there a difference between patients' needs and patients' wants? Think of examples from your own experience of patients' care to illustrate both needs and wants. What are the advantages of giving patients what they need? What are the advantages and disadvantages of giving patients what they want?

Involving all patients in decisions about their care is one of the key aspects of current health service reforms (DOH 2000). The intention is to improve patients' experiences, ensuring that they and professionals make sustainable decisions about where treatment and care will take place and when and how each will be provided.

Over to you

Read Department of Health (2003) *Choice, Responsiveness and Equity in the NHS and Social Care. A National Consultation*, London, DOH. Visit the Department of Health website at www.dh.gov.uk and search for the most recent items on patient choice. With reference to the patient groups for which you provide care:

● What choices do patients/users/carers want?

● What information and support would they need to exercise these choices?

● What changes in the system, or in how people work or communicate, would be needed to create these choices?

● How could these choices be made fair for all?

Establishing priorities and enabling *patient choice* provides a foundation upon which to set goals for care. A goal is a statement about the specific outcome to be achieved as a result of the nursing intervention provided. A *goal* must be measurable, specific, realistic, individualised and indicate a time span within which it will be achieved (Doenges *et al.* 2000). Thus a goal should specify:

Who	Mr Jones
Will do what	will walk to the toilet
Using what means	using a Zimmer frame and accompanied by a health care assistant
To what degree of success	without having to stop and rest
By which date	by 15 December

The nurse then constructs an individualised *action plan* of nursing interventions that will facilitate achievement of the goals agreed with the patient. The degree of success can later be evaluated in the light of experience. The various components of the goal allow for measurable outcomes in relation to several different aspects of a goal. For example, Mr Jones may achieve his walk to the toilet twice a day even if the Zimmer frame proves unsuitable as an aid. Thus goals may be achieved in entirety or partially. In monitoring patient goals the nurse must continually consider:

- the level at which each goal has been set; goals that are achieved very easily may improve the patient's confidence or raise unrealistic expectations of future progress;
- possible changes in the nature of the patient's problem; for example, if Mr Jones develops a urinary tract infection, walking to the toilet may become more difficult;
- whether achievement of the goal requires the help of other professionals such as the physiotherapist or the continence advisor;

Key points Top tips

- Care planning should be undertaken in partnership with the patient when at all possible.
- Partnership is intended to foster concordance rather than compliance.
- Negotiating with patients and enabling them to make choices lays the foundation for the development of individual goals.
- Goals must be measurable, realistic, individualised and time limited.
- A goal should specify who will do what, using what means, to what degree of success, by an agreed date.

- whether to continue until the date on which the goal is to be reviewed or whether to reassess the situation and negotiate a new goal with the patient (Roper *et al.* 2000).

Conclusion

This chapter has helped you to examine critically theoretical ideas about nursing within the context of the nursing process. It has introduced you to associated concepts such as nursing diagnosis and the ways in which this contributes to the formation of goals. Structured approaches to setting goals will enable you to plan and evaluate individualised care for your patients.

RRRRR*Rapid recap*

1 What are the phases of the nursing process?
2 Successful completion of an assessment is dependent upon which factors?
3 Name and describe the five elements that form the basis of the Roper, Logan and Tierney model of assessment.
4 Define a nursing diagnosis.
5 What are the components of a nursing goal?

References

Apple, A. L. and Malcolm, P. (1999) 'The struggle for recognition: the nurse practitioner in New South Wales, Australia', *Clinical Nurse Specialist* 13 (5) pp. 236–41.

Carpenito-Moyet, L. J. (2004) *Handbook of Nursing Diagnosis*, 10th edn. Philadelphia PA, Lippincott, Williams and Wilkins.

Chinn, P. and Kramer, M. K. (2004) *Integrated Knowledge Development in Nursing*, 6th edn. St Louis MO, Mosby.

Department of Health (DOH) (2000) *The NHS Plan. A Plan for Investment. A Plan for Reform*. London, DOH.

Department of Health (DOH) (2003) *Choice, Responsiveness and Equity in the NHS and Social Care. A National Consultation*. London, DOH.

Doenges, M., Moorhouse, M. F. and Burley, J. (2000) *Application of Nursing Process and Nursing Diagnosis: An Interactive Text for Diagnostic Reasoning*. Philadelphia PA, F. A. Davis.

Fawcett, J. (2000) *Analysis and Evaluation of Contemporary Nursing Knowledge: Nursing Models and Theories*, 2nd edn. Philadelphia PA, F. A. Davis.

Gidlow, A. and Ellis, B. (2003) 'Advanced nursing practice and the interface with medicine in the UK', Chapter 13 in P. McGee and G. Castledine (eds) *Advanced Practice*, 2nd edn. Oxford, Blackwell Science, pp. 157–68.

Levine, M. (1966a) 'Adaptation and assessment: a rationale for nursing intervention', *American Journal of Nursing* 66 p. 2450.

Levine, M. (1966b) 'Trophicognosis: an alternative to nursing diagnosis', *American Nurses Association Regional Clinical Conferences* 2 pp. 55–70.

Levine, M. (1967) 'The four conservation principles of nursing', *Nursing Forum* 6 p. 45.

Levine, M. (1969) *Introduction to Clinical Nursing*. Philadelphia PA, F. A. Davis.

McGee, P. (2003) 'International perspectives on advanced nursing practice', Chapter 12 in P. McGee and G. Castledine (eds) *Advanced Practice*, 2nd edn. Oxford, Blackwell Science, pp. 144–56.

Marriner Tomey, A. and Alligood, M. R. (eds) (2002) *Nursing Theorists and Their Work*, 5th edn. St Louis MO, Mosby.

North American Nursing Diagnosis Association (NANDA) (1990) *Taxonomy of Nursing Diagnosis*. St Louis MO, NANDA.

Peplau, H. (1952) *Interpersonal Relations in Nursing*. New York, G. P. Putnam.

Roper, N., Logan, W. and Tierney, A. (2000) *The Roper-Logan-Tierney Model of Nursing: Based on Acitivities of Living*. Edinburgh, Churchill Livingstone.

Schaefer, K. M. (2002) 'Myra Estrin Levine. The conservation model', Chapter 14 in A. Marriner Tomey and M. R. Alligood (eds) *Nursing Theorists and Their Work*, 5th edn. St Louis MO, Mosby, pp. 212–25.

4

Secondary care

Learning outcomes

By the end of this chapter you should be able to:

● briefly explain the concept of direct nursing care and identify the nursing care activities associated with this;

● briefly explain the concept of indirect nursing care;

● develop an understanding of the ways in which nurses may engage in indirect care and the responsibilities associated with this;

● develop an understanding of the role of the environment in nursing care.

Introduction

The term *secondary care* is used to refer to those settings in which patients with complex and emergency needs can receive high levels of technical or specialist treatment and care from members of a wide variety of health disciplines working in one place. Secondary care settings provide opportunities for senior and experienced members of different professions to work together to provide interventions that cannot take place in patients' homes or in their local health centres for reasons that are either practical, financial or a mixture of both. Nursing occupies a pivotal role in secondary care as the only profession that provides continuous, 24-hour services to all patients, a factor that challenges the profession to appraise critically both the nature of care in this context and the environments in which it is delivered. Those patients may be highly dependent on others for assistance in performing all or most of the activities of living (Roper *et al.* 2000) and require additional specialist and technical nursing skills to compensate for deficits in essential body functions. Others may require partial assistance as well as additional expertise and, in some instances, education to enable them to live independently (Orem 2001).

Over to you

How might these three types of nursing intervention described by Orem (2001) relate to nursing in your field of practice?

Which activities compensate for patients' inability to perform daily living activities for themselves?

Which activities provide partial assistance?

Which activities could be classified as educative?

This text will help you: Orem, D. (2001) *Nursing: Concepts of Practice,* 6th edn. St Louis MO, C. V. Mosby.

⊶ᴛ *Keywords*

Direct care

Nursing interventions provided
by a nurse for a particular
patient. Examples of direct
care include performing a bed
bath or mouth care,
administering medication,
dressing a wound, teaching a
patient and carrying out
technical procedures, for
example blood sugar
monitoring or cardiac
massage.

Secondary care settings challenge nurses to appraise critically the
metaparadigm of nursing in relation to the nature of the patients
and their particular health problems. The object of this appraisal is
the provision of sound, evidence-based care. This chapter will help
you to undertake this appraisal through an examination of the needs
of patients in relation to two key concepts about care: **direct** and
indirect care. Inherent in both these concepts is a range of
nursing activities that will help you to clarify the nature of nursing
in secondary care settings and create links with current health
policies, especially those relating to infection control. This particular
topic will help you examine the fourth element of the
metaparadigm, that of the environment and the interplay between
this and nursing.

Direct and indirect care

The concepts of direct and indirect care refer to the type of
engagement that individual practitioners may have with a particular
patient (Koetters 1989). Examining care in this way enables us to
appreciate that care has two dimensions: the overt, hands-on
activities performed by an individual nurse working with a specific
patient; and the tacit roles undertaken by others who may have little
or no patient contact.

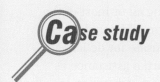

Case study

Staff Nurse Williams has been qualified for about six months and has been
assigned to care for a small group of six patients throughout his span of duty,
beginning at 7.30 a.m. He will be responsible for all the care given to these
patients and will have help from a health care assistant if necessary. After receiving
a handover report from the night staff, he visits each patient in turn to make a quick
assessment of each person's needs and then begins to plan his work. The first
patient, Mr Smith, is unconscious following a head injury sustained during a fight in
a public house during the previous night. He requires regular neurological
observations, pressure area care and attention to personal hygiene. He has several
facial cuts and his hair is matted with blood. An intravenous infusion is in progress.
Members of the medical staff are expected to assess him later in the morning and
request several investigations to ascertain the extent of the injury sustained. Mr
Donovan, the second patient, has been unconscious for several weeks after falling
sixty feet from scaffolding on the building site where he worked. He also requires
pressure area care, attention to personal hygiene, mouth care and passive
movements. His conscious level requires regular monitoring and he needs some
mental stimulation. Parenteral feeding is in progress. The physiotherapist will visit
him later in the morning. The third patient, Mr Jones, 23 years old, broke his leg
playing football at the weekend. He has traction in place and is confined to bed.
He is able to wash himself and attend to his own personal hygiene. He refuses to

allow the female nurses to check his sacral area for any signs of redness and has not had his bowels open for several days as he feels embarrassed at having to use a bedpan. Mr Ali, the fourth patient, was also admitted last night after being knocked down by a car while crossing the road at a pedestrian crossing. He was heavily concussed as a result and he has severe bruising down the right side of his body. He is in a lot of pain. This morning he is worried because he did not remember to tell anyone in the Accident and Emergency (A&E) Department that he has diabetes that is controlled by diet and tablets. The fifth patient, Mr Ravinder Singh Dhillon, is an elderly man with Parkinson's disease. He was admitted yesterday for assessment, as his medication did not seem to be helping. He needs help with almost every activity. During the next few days the medical staff, speech therapist, physiotherapist and occupational therapist will assess him. The final patient is Mr Walker, who is recovering from injuries sustained during an assault at work. He was beaten around the head and trunk, causing fractures to his skull, cheekbones and ribs. He is now able to attend to his own personal hygiene but has a lot of pain and still experiences flashbacks from the assault.

1   What direct care activities will Staff Nurse Williams perform for each patient?
2   What other direct nursing care activities may be required? Which types of nurses should provide these?
3   What is Staff Nurse Williams' role with regard to the care given by other nurses and members of other professional groups?

Direct care refers to those activities in which the nurse delivers care directly to the patient. Direct care may be continuous, that is, delivered by the same primary nurse throughout a shift. Alternatively, direct care may be episodic. For example, a specialist nurse might be asked to provide a more effective pain regimen for Mr Walker or to temporarily take over the care of Mr Smith if a crisis develops as the result of his head injury. Staff Nurse Williams and his immediate colleagues may also have opportunities to learn from more experienced or specialist practitioners who take advantage of their time with his patients to demonstrate their skills or to explain their work to both him and the patient concerned.

An examination of direct care reveals that nursing is a practical and interpersonal activity in which the nurse can consciously adopt specific roles depending on the needs of the patient. In caring for his six patients Staff Nurse Williams may act as a physical carer, negotiator, companion, culture broker, co-ordinator, specialist and technician (McGee 1998).

As a *physical carer* Staff Nurse Williams will either perform certain activities of living for those who cannot do this for themselves or find ways in which to assist those who have difficulty. Mr Smith and Mr Donovan are unconscious and so Staff Nurse Williams will wash, dress and shave both of them and ensure that their mouths are kept clean. He will also clean them and change the bed linen when they are incontinent. Both men will need changes of position every two hours to prevent the formation of pressure sores and, in Mr Donovan's case, passive movements to prevent muscle wastage. The safety of both men is a very important part of physical care as neither is able to prevent himself from falling out of bed, choking or coping with any other hazard. In contrast, patients such as Mr Walker and Mr Jones appear to require far less care. However, the experience of pain may still make it difficult for Mr Walker to cope with certain daily activities unaided. Similarly, Mr Jones may also experience pain and the restricted movement afforded by the traction may make it difficult for him to do everything for himself.

Reflective activity

Everyone is motivated towards self-care. Nurses should only perform care when the patient is unable to do so by reason of illness, injury or disability. The ability to care for oneself is an important indicator of the patient's potential for coping with daily life at home.

There is no such thing as self-care in hospital. Patients who are labelled as self-caring by ward staff are simply neglected. If they were truly able to self-care, patients would not be in hospital.

Think about these two positions in relation to your own place of work.

As a *negotiator* Staff Nurse Williams will work with patients, trying to see situations from their perspectives. This involves assessing what is normal for an individual and identifying how things have changed as a basis for negotiating nursing interventions (Roper *et al.* 2000). For example, Mr Jones is clearly unhappy about certain aspects of his care that he finds embarrassing, particularly when his carers are women. Nurses have a responsibility to ensure that he does not develop sacral sores, but negotiating skills could help both him and the nurses to find a satisfactory solution in which his dignity is not compromised. An explanation of the importance of checking the sacral area twice daily would help him to understand why this task needs to be done and perhaps, with the aid of a mirror, he might be able to do this for himself, for at least some of the time. Mr Dhillon is elderly and, in addition to his Parkinson's disease, may have other disabilities such as hearing loss or visual impairment. He is also to be assessed by a number of different professionals, which could be a tiring and potentially confusing experience. In these circumstances it would be easy for Mr Dhillon's preferences and wishes regarding his long-term care to be overlooked and it is Staff Nurse Williams' responsibility to ensure that this does not occur by discussing Mr Dhillon's preferences with him, supporting him in his discussions with professionals and by advocating on Mr Dhillon's behalf if he so wishes.

In acting as a *companion* Staff Nurse Williams provides a source of social contact for patients. In this context nurse and patient meet as two human beings and can get to know one another in a social medium. Such interaction helps to provide a bond through which interpersonal therapeutic skills can be channelled. For example, Mr Ali is concussed and obviously very worried about managing his diabetes. His first contact with Staff Nurse Williams is likely to be at a social level. The success of that encounter will influence how the information about Mr Ali's diabetes is taken up and whether he feels confident that it will be acted upon. Mr Dhillon may well be feeling very depressed about the effects of his Parkinson's disease. In acting as a companion, the nurse is able to provide encouragement and support throughout his assessment period. Both Mr Smith and Mr Donovan are unconscious but may still be able to hear what is happening around them and to understand what is said to them. In acting as a companion, the nurse is able to provide much-needed stimulation and reassurance that may assist the recovery of full consciousness.

At a deeper level the role of companion allows the nurse privileged insight into patients' lives in ways that are not possible in other types of relationship, even with those to whom we are very close. Companionship leads inevitably to a state of involvement that affords the opportunity to be with patients as they experience the suffering caused by their conditions as well as the good days when their symptoms recede. This involvement allows nurses to learn from patients about aspects of care that cannot be formally taught but which are, nevertheless, crucial to the development of good practice. Involvement also allows nurses to '*presence*' themselves with patients, that is to say, nurses develop a heightened sense of awareness and communication with patients, becoming 'in tune' with those for whom they care (Benner and Wrubel 1989; Benner 1984). The 'presenced' nurse is able to draw on personal qualities and experience that facilitate empathy with patients, anticipation of their needs and the ability to be with them through what may be painful and distressing events. Even if there is nothing that the nurse can do to change those events, his or her presence with the patient provides comfort and support. Such engagement with other people requires a high level of self-awareness and understanding as well as the ability to relate effectively to others, a state that is sometimes referred to as the **therapeutic use of self** (Travelbee 1971).

⊶ 🔑 Keywords

Therapeutic use of self

Consciously drawing on one's own personality and experience and using these to establish relationships with patients through which effective nursing interventions can be applied.

As a *culture broker* Staff Nurse Williams ensures that care is designed and delivered in a way that takes account of each individual patient's cultural values and beliefs. Mr Dhillon's name indicates that his background is Sikh. Mr Ali's name suggests that he may be Muslim. In both instances Staff Nurse Williams will need to check whether they have any particular preferences, especially in relation to whether they wish to engage in religious practices such as prayer or dietary rules. Nursing care can then be planned in one of three ways. First, care may be provided solely within the patient's own culture. Thus, if Mr Ali requests halal food, this can be provided in a way that will meet the requirements of his diabetes. Second, it may be necessary to enable patients to incorporate changes into their lifestyles in ways that are culturally acceptable. If, for example, Mr Ali now requires insulin therapy, then dosages and timing of injections will need to be fitted in with his daily routine. Finally, care may be directed towards helping patients cope with imposed changes. For example, Mr Walker may have to adapt to long-term dependence on others for help when the pain becomes too intense. Depending on his background, there may be culturally based ideas about who he can ask for help and what others may do for him (Leininger and McFarland 2002).

As a *co-ordinator* of care, Staff Nurse Williams acts as a focal point for other disciplines involved in meeting patients' needs. In addition to the medical staff, all Staff Nurse Williams' patients are likely to receive care from physiotherapists. Mr Dhillon may also be assessed by a speech therapist if he has difficulties with swallowing or controlling the flow of saliva, and by an occupational therapist to ascertain his ability to cope at home. Mr Walker may require help from a psychologist in coping with the flashbacks. Staff Nurse Williams is responsible for knowing which therapist is due to visit each patient and when the visits are likely to take place so that care can be planned in ways that allow patients time to rest and eat meals in peace. As each therapist arrives the staff nurse should make sure that he speaks to the individual concerned before therapy begins, passing on relevant information about the patient's health situation. Before each therapist leaves the staff nurse should ensure that he is aware of the interventions provided and any activities that are to be carried out by the ward staff until the therapist is able to call again. Thus the staff nurse acts as the lynch pin, acting in the patient's interests to ensure that therapy is delivered as appropriate and collating information from multiple sources.

As a *technician* Staff Nurse Williams uses technical skills and knowledge to provide, enhance or facilitate treatment for the benefit of patients. This may include the use of an aseptic technique to clean and dress Mr Smith's cuts and to manage his intravenous infusion and Mr Donovan's feeding regime. In addition, Staff Nurse Williams will perform and record neurological observations on Mr Smith and Mr Ali and ensure that Mr Jones's traction is cleaned and positioned correctly.

After only six months of qualified nursing practice Staff Nurse Williams will not yet have had time to develop specialist knowledge and skill. Consequently, he will rely for guidance on more experienced practitioners who have undertaken more advanced courses. These *specialist* nurses provide intermittent episodes of care in relation to specific areas of patient need. For example, Mr Donovan will require the expertise of a nutrition nurse specialist who has undergone post-registration education in order to develop an extended knowledge and skill base in meeting the nutritional needs of patients who are unable to eat. Similarly, Mr Walker and Mr Ali may both require episodes of care from a nurse specialising in pain management. Mr Donovan, Mr Jones and, if he does not regain consciousness, Mr Smith may all require care from a nurse specialising in tissue viability in order to prevent the formation of pressure sores. Mr Ali may also require specialist help in protecting his bruised skin from further deterioration and help from the diabetes nurse specialist in managing his diabetes. In addition to their role in giving episodic direct care, all of these nurses will advise, teach and guide less experienced colleagues such as Staff Nurse Williams, thus enabling them to enhance their own knowledge and skills and provide care in between the specialists' visits.

These direct care activities contrast strongly with those of **indirect care**, which is characterised by lack of contact between

Keywords

Indirect care

Nursing interventions provided by a nurse who has no direct contact with the patient. Examples of indirect care include participation in standard setting or the design of procedures, providing education and training, clinical supervision and acting as a consultant.

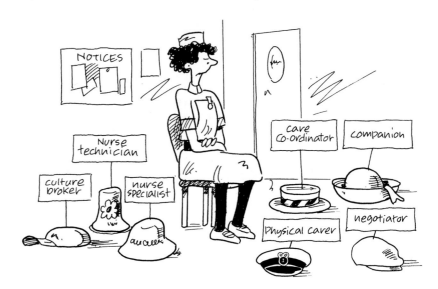

the care provider and the recipient. Indirect care may be continuous in that some providers, such as senior nurse managers and nurse teachers, may have no direct patient contact as a regular part of their jobs but nevertheless contribute through education, supervision and activities directed towards ensuring that standards of care are satisfactory. Alternatively, indirect care may be episodic. For example, Staff Nurse Williams may contact staff in another ward for advice about aids that may help Mr Dhillon to either feed himself or take oral fluids despite his Parkinsonian tremor. The staff consulted may never meet Mr Dhillon but may nevertheless be regarded as having contributed to his care indirectly.

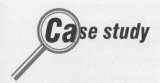

Case study

Eloise Fletcher is the modern matron of the medical ward directorate. Her role has two dimensions. First, she must provide a visible and accessible point of contact for patients and relatives, ensuring that communications between them and the staff are satisfactory and that patients are satisfied with their treatment and care. This aspect of her role requires her to visit each ward at least once every day and speak to every patient to ensure that all is well. Eloise has been on leave for a week and is in the process of making her first round of the patients. On entering ward 4 she finds that Mrs Duffy, who was admitted earlier in the day for an angiogram, is preparing to discharge herself. She tells Eloise 'When they showed me to my bed, there was this white stuff all over the floor. I assumed it was talcum powder and that someone would come and clean it up. I dropped something on the floor and when I looked closely it wasn't talc at all. It was skin. It's disgusting. I'm not staying here.'

Dealing with this situation requires that Eloise first listens to Mrs Duffy and tries to ascertain whether there is any way she can be persuaded to stay for the angiogram that she clearly needs. In addition, she must use the second aspect of her role to provide leadership, for the ward manager and staff, to ensure that they understand the importance of ward cleaning, to identify and rectify whatever shortcomings in the system allowed the situation to occur and do so within the context of a no-blame culture.

Later in the day Eloise attends a matrons' meeting at which she is informed that infection control is now a priority in hospitals. The aim is to tackle the problem of *nosocomial* or hospital-acquired infection, in particular methicillin-resistant staphylococcus aureus (MRSA) (DOH 2004). The matrons discuss ways in which improvements can be made in infection control. The wards have to function within their allocated budgets and staffing levels and it is unlikely that there will be any new funding available to help. The matrons must, therefore, find ways of working with staff to enable them to achieve what is required. A suggestion is made to include the nurse consultants and staff in the clinical governance department. The matrons agree that approaches will be made to enlist support from both sources.

On returning to her office, Eloise phones Louise Fry, the nurse consultant in her directorate. The two work very closely together and meet every week to discuss their work. They agree to meet tomorrow to plan a strategy for infection control.

1   What types of indirect nursing care activities can you identify?

2   How would you improve infection control in your workplace?

Analysis of events in any hospital ward will show that, in addition to the direct care activities, there is a wide range of indirect nursing work that also contributes to patient well-being. Some of this work requires the same skills as those used in direct care, but used in different ways. Other aspects of indirect care reveal nursing roles that may not be apparent in face-to-face encounters between nurses and patients but which nevertheless carry the same professional responsibility and accountability as direct care activities (NMC 2002). In fulfilling her role as modern matron (DOH 2001a), Eloise may act as leader, negotiator, empowerer, teacher, specialist and manager.

As *leader*, Eloise is required to develop a vision of what is to be achieved and, using expert interpersonal communication skills, to share that vision with the ward managers and staff. Her **democratic leadership** style will provide opportunities for staff to express their views, make contributions and ask questions, thus becoming involved in the process of change. As the clinical leader, her colleague Louise, the nurse consultant, has a different style. For her, a **transformational leadership** style is directed towards motivating and encouraging ward managers and staff to share the vision of what is to be achieved by encouraging them to question and challenge the ideas presented until these are expressed 'in a language that they understand and that appeals to their professional values and beliefs' (Close 2003 p. 64). Between them, Eloise and Louise will provide a flexible form of leadership that enables others to feel part of what is happening and that is intended to 'help others to grow and to encourage them toward self actualisation [by] competent, caring leaders who are interested in the success and well-being of their followers' (Hanson and Malone 2000 p. 290).

A *negotiator* uses interpersonal skills to resolve challenging situations. Both Eloise's and Louise's roles require them to deal directly with the concerns of patients and relatives and to do whatever they can to rectify deficiencies in the care and services. In this context, they must listen empathetically to complaints and worries that may be expressed very emotionally and be seen to act on the issues raised.

Keywords

Democratic leadership

A people oriented approach in which those who are led have the opportunity to participate in discussion about what is to be achieved and in subsequent decision making. Power is thus shared, in contrast to autocratic leadership in which the leader retains all authority and tells others what to do.

Transformational leadership

A process in which leaders and followers work together to create shared goals and work collaboratively towards these. Transformational leadership raises followers' aspirations and enables them to achieve their own goals (Marriner Tomey 1993).

Reflective activity

How many complaints have been made in your ward or department in the last six months?

What do patients complain about and why?

How did staff respond when a complaint was made?

Both Eloise and Louise must also be able to negotiate with nursing staff and other colleagues about all aspects of delivering care, developing or changing services in ways that reflect cultural competence, a term that in this instance refers to their understanding of the organisation in which they work, how it functions, and the personalities and relationships involved. Organisational culture can be described as 'the way we do things around here', and understanding of this culture will facilitate negotiation (Birnbaum and Somers 1986). Becoming culturally competent also requires Eloise and Louise to think politically. Both are in positions in which they can influence nursing and other colleagues by working with them, contributing to the development of strategies and working together to develop standards, in this case for infection control.

In her role as *empowerer* Eloise enables members of the nursing staff to clarify their understanding and expectations in relation to infection control and encourages them to take the lead in reviewing and developing their practice. This could be achieved through *clinical practice benchmarking*. This concept arises from total quality management:

> a corporate business management philosophy which recognises that customer needs and business goals are inseparable. It is applicable within both industry and commerce. It ensures maximum effectiveness and efficiency within a business and secures commercial leadership by putting in place processes and systems which promote excellence, prevent errors and ensure that every aspect of the business is aligned to customer needs.
>
> (Pike and Barnes 1996 p. 24)

Setting standards is part of 'processes and systems'. To assist in this there is a range of quality management standards that provide a yardstick against which to test our own processes and systems. These are produced by the British Standards Institution and cover products/services, environmental matters and management systems. Benchmarking is one of the processes through which quality is determined in a particular service or aspect of care (Gilbert 1994).

Clinical practice benchmarking has been introduced as part of current health service reforms intended to improve the quality of care by making it everyone's responsibility (Ellis 2000). Achieving quality rests in part on effective leadership but also on the setting and monitoring of standards based on the best available evidence to support practice. Emphasis is placed on eliminating poor performance and learning from mistakes. In this context clinical practice benchmarking has become 'a process through which best practice is identified and continuous improvement pursued through comparison and sharing' (DOH 1999 p. 49) (see Figure 4.1). The *Essence of Care* document (DOH 2001b) introduced benchmarking for eight nursing care activities (see Figure 4.2). Each care activity is addressed in a series of steps. First, a nursing team meets to identify concerns about a care activity that requires standards and benchmarking. Second, important factors in establishing best practice are examined. These include an evaluation of the evidence that underpins current practice and that is available to inform further development. Evidence may be drawn from research, expert opinion and other sources. Third, good practice is graded using an agreed scale. Fourth, the team then make contact with another nursing team working in the same field of practice and compare steps one to three. Finally, the original team is able to agree and set standards that are monitored and reviewed at intervals by repeating steps one to four.

- Focuses attention on both the quantifiable and the non-quantifiable aspects of care.
- Is consistent with the development of a blame-free workplace culture.
- Enables practitioners to justify best practice with reference to the best available evidence.

- Incorporates a 'window on the world' outside the immediate working environment.
- Incorporates users' views.
- Facilitates sharing and dissemination of good practice.
- Does not provide a 'once and for all' standard but facilitates improvement through audit and monitoring procedures.

Figure 4.1 *Advantages of benchmarking*

- Personal and oral hygiene
- Privacy and dignity
- Pressure ulcers
- Continence and bladder and bowel care

- Food and nutrition
- Safety of people with mental illness
- Record keeping
- Principles of self-care

Figure 4.2 *Care activities for clinical practice benchmarking*

👉 *Over to you*

Read Wilkin, K. (2003) 'The meaning of caring in the practice of intensive care nursing', *British Journal of Nursing* 12 (20) pp. 1178–85. To what extent could the ideas about care identified here be benchmarked?

As a *teacher* Eloise provides education for nursing staff in ways that facilitate learning that can be translated into practice. She may undertake some of this education herself if she feels that she has the appropriate knowledge base but, as the modern matron, she may find that her time is limited. However, she is responsible for ensuring that members of staff have appropriate opportunities and resources for learning. In contrast, the nurse consultant has a specific role in teaching and guiding nurses (Spross *et al.* 2000). Eloise and Louise may work together to plan a programme for staff about improvements in infection control.

Specialists undertake and utilise post-registration education in a specific area of patient care, such as stoma care, continence advice, pain management or diabetes management. If Eloise has undertaken such education she will be able to act as a resource, advising and supervising staff in the development of this aspect of their practice. Alternatively she may invite other nurses, such as those working in infection control, to work with staff in the directorate in order to bring about change.

> ### Over to you
>
> Look up post-registration courses in your field of practice. Which courses are available and what topics do they cover? How might completing such a course help you to achieve your career goals?

Eloise's role as modern matron is rooted in *management* and the notion of hierarchy. Her position requires that she achieve specified targets through the implementation of Trust policies and procedures, setting objectives for staff, planning and organising work in ways that facilitate the attainment of particular goals. Staff wanting to introduce any changes will need to ensure that they present their case in a way that matches the targets that Eloise has been given in order to convince both her and her superiors that their proposals are a useful contribution. Failure to do so will usually mean that their ideas are rejected or ignored. In contrast, Louise, as a nurse consultant, is free from managerial responsibilities. Most of her time is spent in the clinical area working directly with staff and patients, providing leadership in practice, professional advice and education and undertaking research when needed (DOH 1999).

- Nurses may provide care directly or indirectly.
- Both types of care carry professional responsibilities.
- Direct care involves specific activities: physical carer, negotiator, companion, culture broker; co-ordinator, technician and specialist.
- Providing direct care allows the nurse to engage in the therapeutic use of self.
- Indirect care involves leadership, negotiation, empowerment of others, teaching, specialist skills and management;
- Modern matrons and nurse consultants are examples of new senior nursing roles that carry responsibilities for the standards of care.
- Clinical practice benchmarking is a process through which nursing teams can:
  - identify areas of care in which standards are needed;
  - evaluate available evidence;
  - develop, implement and monitor agreed standards of care.

Creating an environment for nursing

Examination of senior nursing roles such as those of modern matron or nurse consultant helps to illustrate the interplay between nursing and the environment. Nurse theorists argue that the environment is a key element of the metaparadigm for nursing, taking the view that the settings in which people live, work or socialise can have positive or negative effects on their health (Fawcett 2000). The internal environment of the person is subject to physiological and psychological changes that may be caused by the environment or, alternatively, impact on the individual's ability to function appropriately.

One of the noticeable features of nursing theories is that, while they are all based on the metaparadigm of nursing, few address the environment in which nursing care takes place. This seems rather a serious omission when we consider the interrelationship between the environment and nursing work. At a physical level, the geography of any hospital ward will influence the ways in which the nursing staff organise their work. The most ill patients are likely to be situated nearest to the nurses' station. The location of the linen store, sluice and bathrooms may all influence the way in which care is organised to minimise the need for too many trips up and down the ward. The Trust will create a work environment in which policies and procedures are formulated and publicised to make clear what the organisation expects from staff. Professional groups within

---

> ### Over to you
>
> Compare and contrast the ideas of Nightingale, Orem, Roy and Roper about the environment in relation to the following:
>
> Summarise the key points that each theorist makes about the environment.
>
> 1 Which theorists regard the person as passive, waiting for the environment to act on him/her?
>
> 2 Which theorists regard the person as active, able to act on his/her environment?
>
> 3 What are your ideas about the nature of the environment and the impact that it may have on people's health?
>
> The following resources will help you:
>
> Nightingale, F. (1860/1969) *Notes on Nursing: What It Is and What It Is Not.* New York, Dover Publications.
>
> Orem, D. (2001) *Nursing: Concepts of Practice,* 6th edn. St Louis MO, C. V. Mosby.
>
> Roper, N., Logan, W. and Tierney, A. (2000) *The Roper-Logan-Tierney Model of Nursing: Based on Activities of Living.* Edinburgh, Churchill Livingstone.
>
> Roy, C. and Andrews, H. (1999) *The Roy Adaptation Model.* Stamford CT, Appleton Lange.

the Trust will set standards to which practitioners are expected to adhere. In each ward, the nursing team will create a social sub-culture based on members' attitudes to their work, each other, their patients and the hierarchy that dictates who has the power to make decisions. It is, therefore, essential to create the right environment for nurses to provide care. While there may be little that can be done to change the physical aspects of a care setting, it is the organisational and social elements that usually have most influence

---

> ### Reflective activity
>
> Consider the following questions in relation to two places you have worked recently:
>
> 1 How did staff treat one another?
>
> 2 What was the relationship like between staff and managers?
>
> 3 What activities were routine?
>
> 4 How did staff feel about their work?
>
> 5 Were there any rituals, traditions or symbols in regular use?
>
> 6 Who was regarded as a hero/heroine and why?
>
> 7 How receptive were the team to change?

on whether nurses feel able to give good quality care. The following questions will help you to appraise critically the environment in which care takes place.

How did staff treat one another?

The first question in the last activity asks us to consider what it is like to belong to a team. In ward A, staff are friendly and respect one another as professionals, and each makes a contribution to patient care. They value each other's opinion and the work that each performs. They feel they can rely on each other, helping each other to get through the workload, which is very heavy. Problems do arise. Sometimes people forget to do things or do not do what is expected, but the ward manager, or his deputy, quickly addresses these matters by either discussing them directly with the individual concerned or, if appropriate, raising them in an anonymous way at a staff meeting. The ward manager and deputy are very approachable and understand the strengths and weaknesses of their staff members, none of whom want to be thought of as letting their colleagues down. In contrast, in ward B staff do not get on together very well. Medical staff verbally abuse the nurses, telling them that they are incompetent and useless. The ward manager does nothing to challenge this behaviour and nurses feel resentful. They rarely talk to each other unless absolutely necessary. Staff turnover is very high.

Working as a team is an important part of nursing. Patient care is too complex for one person to do all that is required and, even if that were possible, we still need our colleagues for support and encouragement. Creating a positive team atmosphere helps staff to feel that they are valued, doing something worthwhile in which they can take pride. Mistakes, if they occur, should be dealt with appropriately so that staff are not humiliated or embarrassed.

What was the relationship like between staff and managers?

This question asks us to think about the ways in which the team interacts with non-members. In ward A the staff, the ward manager and his deputy know one another well. They socialise at break times and ask each other's opinions about patient care and ward organisation. The ward manager spends time getting to know his staff both in terms of their professional experience and expertise as well as their personal circumstances. He knows the names of their immediate family members and staff confide in him when problems arise at home. When staff first join the ward team he makes clear his expectations of them. The ward manager has cultivated a similar relationship with more senior nurse managers. The managers work as a team in a similar way to the ward staff. Management decisions are made as a team following consultation with staff. In ward B the turnover of staff is high and thus the ward manager has little time to get to know her staff well. Her manner towards them is rather distant and she does not believe in socialising with staff, arguing that it is not possible to be a friend and a manager at the same time. The ward manager does not get on well with the senior nurse managers, whose attitude to their work is one of 'let's do it to them (patients, doctors, staff, anybody) before they do it to us', which is reflected in their confrontational styles of interaction.

Working as a team extends beyond the confines of the hospital ward. Good relations between managers and staff are based on mutual respect and recognition that each party is contributing to patient care in different ways. A team approach to decision making following consultation means that no one individual is responsible for popular or unpopular decisions. Consequently everyone can concentrate on the work in hand and feel valued without anyone seeming to outshine the others or become labelled because they made decisions that no one really liked (Hanson and Malone 2000).

What activities were routine?

This question asks us to think about the everyday aspects of working in the team. In ward A the ward manager interviews every new member of staff to explain his expectations, for example about standards of dress, punctuality, standard of work. He also tries to clarify the individual's training needs, ambitions and plans. This interview is followed by an induction programme and the allocation of the new member of staff to a mentor who will help that person to settle in. More informal discussions, both individually and in staff meetings, allow the manager opportunities to get to know his staff well. The normal duties and responsibilities of each staff member are set out in written job descriptions, copies of which are given to each new staff member. Further copies are available in the ward office. The daily workload is dependent on the needs of patients, but the ward manager monitors this to ensure that individuals are not overburdened with too many patients with complex needs or who require considerable effort to move. The ward manager encourages staff to develop professionally through participation in hospital working parties and committees. Individuals undertaking these roles are expected to gather the views of their colleagues and report back in staff meetings about their activities. In ward B written job descriptions are also supplied, and morale is so low that staff feel the safest thing to do is to follow these documents rigidly. They fear that if they do anything not listed in the job description, then the doctors will criticise them publicly. They also know that the ward manager will not support them. Timekeeping in ward B is lax, with some members of staff habitually arriving late or leaving early, especially on the late and night shifts. No one seems to know what is happening with the patients and, if asked a question, staff will usually say 'I don't know. I've been on days off.'

Sound effective management is dependent on good relationships between the parties concerned. If managers do not set out what is required, then staff will not know what is expected of them. If staff feel intimidated or unsure of their roles, then they are unlikely to show enthusiasm or initiative in their work. Using excuses such as having been off duty suggests that staff are switched off, do not know and perhaps do not really care about what is happening to their patients

How did staff feel about their work?

This question helps us to explore how it feels to work in a particular environment. In ward A staff feel very positive about their work. They recognise that nursing has a strong hierarchical base, which means that some individuals have higher seniority and sometimes far more responsibility in matters of patient care than do others. However, this does not mean that anyone is preoccupied by status. The sub-culture of ward A allows each member of staff the opportunity to develop their role in ways that enhance their contribution. For example, one of the health care assistants previously worked in mental health and is able to contribute her experience to the care of patients who have attempted suicide. Other members of the ward team value these contributions and incorporate her ideas where it is possible to do so. In ward B the medical staff rule the roost. They regard themselves as the most important people in the Trust, having pioneered new treatments that have attracted both money and good publicity. Nurses are tolerated as necessary but stupid nuisances. Other disciplines are unworthy of their notice.

The status of the work nurses undertake is important. If nurses themselves feel that their efforts are of little value and that they will be dismissed or ridiculed, then they are likely to wonder whether it is worth trying to provide care. Demoralised and abused staff cannot provide care as a positive experience for patients. However, it has to be acknowledged that nurses' greatest enemy in terms of undervaluing their work is their own attitude. The average nurse, when asked about his or her work will shrug and reply 'I am just a staff nurse' or 'We just look after patients when they come back from theatre.' If nurses can dismiss their work so lightly, then it is small wonder that other disciplines see no value in it. Professions such as medicine place much greater value on the expertise and skill of their members, and there is no reason why nurses should not do the same. There is no such thing as being 'just a staff nurse', but there *is* a professional who studies hard for three years to gain his/her initial qualifications and then undertakes additional, more specialised courses. This person is responsible for the welfare of post-operative patients, ensuring, in each case, that respiration and heart rate remain within normal limits, that infusions run on time and that drains are patent. This person knows how to monitor changes in levels of consciousness and how to identify signs of complications such as post-operative haemorrhage. This person also knows what to do if any of these complications arises and may thus be responsible for saving a patient's life.

Were there any rituals, traditions or symbols in regular use?

This question helps us to think about the ways in which the team creates events and traditions that help it function. In ward A the staff meet three times in each 24-hour period for a handover report. This usually takes place in the ward office and is accompanied by a cup of tea. The ward manager argues that this is important because, if staff members are to work as a team, they must have the opportunity to meet each other as team members. Moreover, the workload is so high that quite often the handover report provides the only opportunity for some nurses to have a drink. In ward B the same ritual is in place but only when the ward manager is not around. One nurse is always posted in the ward area as a lookout for any passing senior manager who, it is assumed, will be hostile. The senior nurse managers know about the tea drinking and play cat and mouse in an effort to catch the staff.

Rituals and traditions can be very helpful in building and sustaining a sense of belonging to a team. Provided rituals are not abused, most managers will exercise their professional judgement by turning a blind eye to them. Allowing situations to develop in which managers and staff play games trying to catch one another out does not provide a basis for harmonious working relationships. Similarly, symbols can also be helpful in enabling staff to feel positive about their work, for example changes in uniform to denote seniority, or holding the keys to denote status and a position of trust. Nurses have a long tradition of using symbols to enhance their feelings of self-esteem. By and large, these are harmless but, like the tea drinking in ward B, they can easily be used as weapons in confrontation with managers.

Who was regarded as a hero/heroine and why?

This question asks us to identify those we admire either within the team or among those outside it. Every organisation has members of staff who are regarded as excellent role models. Such role models may be officially sanctioned by the Trust as examples of clinical or professional excellence. However, it is just as likely that heroes/heroines are unofficial; they may be individuals who have done something that their colleagues regard as outstanding or they may have challenged the organisation successfully when others feared to do so, especially when this challenge has involved some sort of confrontation with those who have power.

How receptive were the team to change?

This question asks us to think about whether the team is ready to accept change. In ward B the staff are left to work things out for themselves, a situation that causes stress unless someone decides to help new people informally. Introducing change will be difficult because those who already feel stressed out will not welcome anything new. In contrast, the culture of ward A can enable people to fit in, feel secure and develop a sense of belonging. If people feel secure, they are more likely to cope well with change. However, fitting in is dependent to some extent on communication between the ward manager and other staff so that new recruits can learn what is required of them. If the team is too inward looking, staff may feel very contented with the status quo and be reluctant to change. What matters is the importance of creating an environment in which nursing can flourish to provide optimum care for patients and in which nurses can feel that what they do makes a difference to those who depend on them.

Key points Top tips

- Organisational and social factors play an important part in creating a suitable environment for the provision of care.
- Team leaders/ ward managers play a significant part in creating suitable care environments.
- If members of staff feel secure and valued, they are more likely to use their initiative and actively contribute to patient care beyond the minimum required by their job descriptions.
- Creation of a positive environment for care will facilitate the introduction of change.

Conclusion

This chapter has helped you to examine the concepts of direct and indirect care in hospital settings. Both carry the same professional responsibilities and levels of accountability. Both are dependent on team working in which nursing and nurses feel valued and worthwhile. Bullying and confrontation have no place in creating an environment for care from which patients can benefit, but consideration of the environment for nursing is a neglected aspect of the nursing metaparadigm.

RRRRRRapid recap

1   What is direct care? Give an example.
2   What is indirect care? Give an example.
3   What did Travelbee (1971) mean by therapeutic use of self?
4   Briefly explain the following terms: nurse consultant, modern matron, specialist nurse.
5   Briefly explain the process of clinical practice benchmarking.

References

Benner, P. (1984) *From Novice to Expert. Excellence and Power in Clinical Nursing Practice*. Menlo Park CA, Addison Wesley.

Benner, P. and Wrubel, J. (1989) *The Primacy of Caring. Stress and Coping in Health and Illness*. Menlo Park CA, Addison Wesley.

Birnbaum, D. and Somers, M. (1986) 'The influence of occupational image sub-culture on job attitudes, job performance and job-attitude–job-performance relationship', *Human Relations* 39 (7) pp. 661–72.

Close, A. (2003) 'Supervision and leadership in advanced nursing practice', Chapter 6 in P. McGee and G. Castledine (eds) *Advanced Nursing Practice*, 2nd edn. Oxford, Blackwell Science, pp. 59–72.

Department of Health (DOH) (1999) *Making a Difference. Strengthening the Nursing, Midwifery and Health Visiting Contribution to Health and Healthcare*. London, DOH.

Department of Health (DOH) (2001a) *Implementing the NHS Plan: Modern Matrons. Strengthening the Role of Ward Sisters and Introducing Senior Sisters*, HSC 2001/10.

Department of Health (DOH) (2001b) *The Essence of Care. Patient-focused Benchmarking for Health Care Practitioners*. London, DOH.

Department of Health (DOH) (2004) *A Matron's Charter. An Action Plan for Cleaner Hospitals*. London, DOH.

Ellis, J. (2000) 'Sharing the evidence: clinical practice benchmarking to improve continuously the quality of care', *Journal of Advanced Nursing* 32 (1) pp. 215–25.

Fawcett, J. (2000) *Analysis and Evaluation of Contemporary Nursing Knowledge: Nursing Models and Theories*, 2nd edn. Philadelphia PA, F. A. Davis.

Gilbert, M. (1994) *Understanding Quality Management Standards*. London, Hodder and Stoughton.

Hanson, C. and Malone, B. (2000) 'Leadership: empowerment, change agency and activism', Chapter 10 in A. Hamric, J. Spross and C. Hanson (eds) *Advanced Nursing Practice. An Integrative Approach*, 3rd edn. Philadelphia PA, W. B. Saunders, pp. 279–314.

Koetters, T. (1989) 'Clinical practice and direct patient care', Chapter 5 in A. Hamric and J. Spross (eds) *The Clinical Nurse Specialist in Theory and Practice*, 2nd edn. Philadelphia PA, W. B. Saunders, pp. 107–24.

Leininger, M. and McFarland, M. (2002) *Transcultural Nursing: Concepts, Theories, Research and Practice*, 3rd edn. London, McGraw Hill.

McGee, P. (1998) *Models of Nursing in Practice. A Pattern for Practical Care*. Cheltenham, Nelson Thornes.

Marriner Tomey, A. (1993) *Transformational Leadership in Nursing*. St Louis MO, Mosby Year Book.

Nightingale, F. (1860/1969) *Notes on Nursing: What It Is and What It Is Not*. New York, Dover Publications.

Nursing and Midwifery Council (NMC) (2002) *Code of Professional Conduct*. London, NMC.

Orem, D. (2001) *Nursing: Concepts of Practice*, 6th edn. St Louis MO, C. V. Mosby.

Pike, J. and Barnes, R. (1996) *TQM In Action. A Practical Approach to Continuous Performance Improvement,* 2nd edn. London, Chapman and Hall.

Roper, N., Logan, W. and Tierney, A. (2000) *The Roper-Logan-Tierney Model of Nursing: Based on Activities of Living.* Edinburgh, Churchill Livingstone.

Roy, C. and Andrews, H. (1999) *The Roy Adaptation Model*, Stamford CT, Appleton Lange.

Spross, J., Clarke, E. and Beauregard, J. (2000) 'Expert coaching and guidance', Chapter 7 in A. Hamric, J. Spross and C. Hanson (eds) *Advanced Nursing Practice. An Integrative Approach*, 3rd edn. Philadelphia PA, W. B. Saunders, pp. 183–210.

Travelbee, J. (1971) *Interpersonal Aspects of Nursing*, 2nd edn. Philadelphia PA, F. A. Davis.

Wilkin K. (2003) 'The meaning of caring in the practice of intensive care nursing', *British Journal of Nursing* 12 (20) pp. 1178–85.

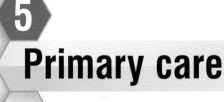

Primary care

Learning outcomes

By the end of this chapter you should be able to:

- briefly explain the importance and usefulness of including health in the nursing metaparadigm;
- demonstrate an understanding of one approach to the management of long-term conditions in primary care settings;
- discuss at least two aspects of health promotion and disease prevention in primary care.

Introduction

The term *primary care* refers to those settings in which patients receive treatment and care within the environment of their own homes or local health centres following consultation with community-based health professionals such as general practitioners and district nurses. Primary care practitioners provide the first point of contact between the National Health Service and those who use it. For the majority of service users this contact will remain at community level because the main focus of primary care roles is to enable people to improve or maintain their health, to diagnose and treat a range of conditions and illness and to refer patients, where necessary, to other sources of help in secondary care.

> ### Over to you
>
> Look up the following terms and make brief notes about each nursing role:
>
> Practice nurse   School nurse
>
> District nurse   Public health nursing
>
> Health visitor

The emphasis on health in the nursing metaparadigm means that nurses are ideally placed to engage in the provision of primary care services. This chapter helps you to examine some of the key aspects of nursing in primary care. It begins with a discussion about the concept of health and why it is important in nursing care. The chapter then provides an opportunity to examine two aspects of health within primary care: caring for patients with long-term health problems and actively promoting health through a range of activities that include screening individuals at risk of developing certain health problems, providing vaccinations and working with patients who are dependent on nicotine.

Health and nursing

Fawcett (2000) states that within the nursing metaparadigm health is concerned with what is normal for each individual and thus provides a basis for a holistic approach to care.

Over to you

Compare and contrast the following definitions of health. Which do you agree or disagree with and why? To what extent are these definitions applicable in primary care?

1   Health is being well, not being ill. What we call disease is 'the reparative process which Nature has instituted' and which is affected by the environment. The environment is the cause of illness. It can also affect the course of an illness. Reference: Nightingale, F. (1860/1969) *Notes on Nursing: What It Is and What It Is Not*. New York, Dover Publications.

2   Health is a dynamic state in which the individual continuously adapts to stress in the internal or external environment in order to maximise potential. Reference: King, I. (1981) *A Theory for Nursing: Systems, Concepts, Processes*. New York, John Wiley and Sons.

3   Health is a dynamic concept in which there is personal growth in the direction of 'creative, constructive, productive, personal and community living'. Reference: Peplau, H. (1952) *Interpersonal Relations in Nursing*. New York, G. P. Putnam. Health is something that is always changing. Health may fail because of a lack of knowledge, resources or a breakdown in the nurse-patient relationship. Health may also fail because professionals cannot organise themselves properly. Reference: Simpson, H. (1991) *Peplau's Model in Action*. Basingstoke, Macmillan.

4   Health is a continuum in which the opposing poles are wellness and illness. Recipients of nursing care, which may be individuals, families or social groups, are composed of systems that incorporate psychological, physiological, sociocultural, developmental and spiritual factors. These systems are in constant interaction with the environment. Consequently, the health continuum is dynamic and subject to change. Wellness is a state in which systems are balanced and working in harmony. Illness is disharmony arising from entropy, a situation in which there is a loss of energy and at the same time disorganisation in or between systems. Reference: Neuman, B. and Fawcett, J. (2002) *The Neuman Systems Model*. Upper Saddle River NJ, Prentice Hall.

In focusing on health, rather than illness, the nurse is able to gain insight into an individual's lifestyle, work and home circumstances and the ways in which these may affect that person's health. In addition, the nurse can develop an understanding of the patient's knowledge and interpretation of a particular illness and the impact this may have on professional attempts to provide help. In this context, illness can be seen as an episode within a life rather than the defining characteristic of that life. Health is, therefore, more than the absence of disease. Health focuses on the quality of life both now and in the future in both positive and negative terms (Close 2003).

There is no single definition of health that suits every aspect of human existence. Nightingale clearly regarded health as the opposite of illness and disease, which, in her view, were caused by the external environment. Her ideas must be seen within the context of her time, when many life-threatening diseases such as cholera, diphtheria and typhoid were caused by external environmental factors. The absence of antibiotics and other modern medicines meant that there was often little that professionals could do other than ensure that patients were as comfortable as possible and hope that Nature, the body's innate healing processes, would enable them to recover. The role of the nurse, as far as Nightingale was concerned, was to ensure that each patient received care that promoted and encouraged the effects of Nature through, for example, physical comfort, cleanliness, rest and nutrition in an environment that had adequate heating, lighting and ventilation. If the environment could cause disease then it could also provide the conditions required for Nature to effect a recovery (Nightingale 1860/1969).

Reflective activity

Select one patient for whom you have provided care at home. To what extent might factors in the environment of that home help or hinder the patient's recovery?

Modern ideas about health look beyond the external environment, drawing on an understanding of the person as not only a physical but also a psychological, social and spiritual being. Health is now regarded as an element of each of these four aspects of the person. It is also a product of the interrelationships between them. Thus illness or disease in one aspect can affect health in some if not all of the others. Health is now understood as a far more complex phenomenon than in Nightingale's day and, consequently, there are many different explanations of what it means.

> ## Over to you
>
> Write down your own definitions of physical health, mental health, social health and spiritual health. Give reasons for your definitions. Compare and contrast your definitions and the reasons for these with those of your colleagues or fellow students.

The World Health Organization (WHO 1946) defined health as a 'state of complete physical, mental and social well-being and not merely the absence of disease and infirmity'. This definition is widely used among health professionals. It appears to incorporate all the aspects of the person and could, therefore, be regarded as a fairly satisfactory and succinct way of summing up the nature of health. However, it is not at all clear what is intended by 'complete physical, mental and social well-being', and it is therefore difficult to know if or how this might be achieved or the criteria by which it could be judged. The term 'well-being' is vague, setting no boundary for the concept of health. Consequently, an individual might be considered unhealthy 'if she is unhappy, or bored, living on her own in a terraced house in Warrington when she wants to be married and living in France' (Seedhouse 1991 p. 47).

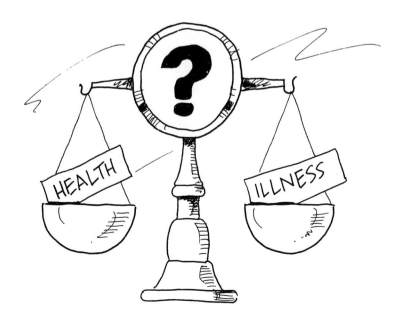

The view of health put forward by WHO suggests that those who are sick or have some form of disability cannot be healthy. This has particular implications for nurses working in primary care settings in that many of their patients will have some form of enduring health problem such as diabetes, asthma or arthritis. Much of the nurses' work will be directed towards helping these patients to manage their health problems in ways that enable them to have active, independent lives. With effective management many will have periods in which they are symptom free and can say that they are 'healthy for me', yet the view implied by WHO is that they cannot possess health if they have a disease. Similarly, those with disabilities are also implicitly incapable of health because they cannot attain the complete state of 'well-being' that this would require.

'Well-being' implies that health is a single state that each person seeks to attain. This idea takes no account of individual differences. If people with enduring health problems or disabilities can be described as healthy, then it follows that their health will in some way differ from the health of those without such conditions. If health is associated with the interrelationships between the physical, psychological, social and spiritual aspects of the person, then it is clear that each individual will have his or her own view and experience of what health means to them. Therefore, health cannot be a single state because each person is unique.

Moreover health is not static. Each person has an internal environment that is constantly changing throughout the day and night in response to physical and psychological processes such as digestion, breathing, the production of waste, thinking and feeling (King 1981). That person also experiences and responds to the external environment, which can be social or physical. Thus the person experiences constant challenges that require some kind of adaptation. This has implications for nurses working in primary care in terms of recognising and facilitating these adaptations that may be beneficial to an individual. Positive adaptations could include encouraging and supporting someone to stop smoking in order to improve their respiratory function or to lose weight in order to reduce breathlessness. Positive adaptations promote harmony within and between the internal and external environments resulting in 'wellness' (Neuman and Fawcett 2002).

Maladaptive responses to challenges result in illness (Neuman and Fawcett 2002). Maladaptation can occur for a number of reasons. Each individual is unique and thus has his or her own degree or level of resilience, resources or motivation to cope with the constant demands of the internal and external environments. In some instances those demands may be so intense that they overwhelm the individual's ability to cope, making adaptation almost impossible. Thus exposure to a harmful substance such as asbestos, the development of cancerous changes in the cells or the experience of a serious traffic accident may incur demands with which the individual just cannot cope. Conceptualising health in terms of adaptation is associated with personal responsibility. The nurse can facilitate and support adaptation but ultimately the responsibility for change is that of the individual concerned. Failure or inability to adapt could, therefore, incur censure.

Key points *Top tips*

- Including health in the metaparadigm of nursing allows the nurse to adopt a holistic approach to the patient rather than just focus on illness or disease.
- There is no completely satisfactory definition of health.
- Every nurse theorist provides a particular view that reflects the time and circumstances in which that nursing theory was developed.
- Health can co-exist, in the same person, with illness, disability or disease.
- Health is best defined by the individual.
- An individual's health is constantly changing.
- Individuals can take action to protect their health but cannot control everything that may affect it.

Peplau (1952) acknowledged the limitations of individuals with regard to maintaining their health. As a psychiatric nurse, Peplau viewed health largely from a psychological and social perspective. In her view, health is about personal development that enables the individual to lead as full a life as possible. In educating, supporting and facilitating patients, the primary care nurse is working towards a similar goal that is inconsistent with blaming or judging patients for their failures. Peplau (1952) is particularly explicit about the importance of the *therapeutic nurse–patient relationship*, which, in her view, differs from other social relationships. The therapeutic relationship has four phases. In the *orientation phase* the nurse and patient meet initially as strangers and must accord each other the courtesies normally afforded to those whom we meet for the first time. They work collaboratively to identify the patient's problems. In the *identification phase* the patient and the nurse identify who can best meet that individual's needs. In the *exploitation phase* the patient makes use of and responds to the professional interventions provided. He or she may be completely dependent on the nurse, be partially dependent on the nurse but independent in some ways or be completely able to function without assistance. The nurse's goal is to help the patient towards such independence and in the final, *resolution phase*, the nurse–patient relationship is brought to a close (Peplau 1952; Howk 2002). Thus the therapeutic relationship is one that has a defined purpose: to be of benefit to the patient, and of a limited duration, ending as the patient achieves independence, all of which are inconsistent with blaming people who cannot adapt successfully to changes in the environment.

Reflective activity

Compare and contrast Peplau's four stages of the nurse–patient relationship with the modern concept of the nursing process outlined on p. 37.

In Peplau's view, nursing is a maturing force that requires professionals to confront aspects of human existence that the majority of people never have to consider or wish to consider in themselves or in others (Peplau 1952). The kind of person that the nurse is, and becomes, through the experience of caring for patients, has direct implications for the type of therapeutic relationships that individuals will establish and the ways in which patients may benefit from the care that follows (Howk 2002). Nursing therefore requires practitioners to become aware of their own values and beliefs, the ways in which they interact with others, and how these may enhance or detract from the therapeutic relationship (Campinha-Bacote 2003). Nowhere in nursing is this more important than when working alone with patients in the privacy of their homes. In these circumstances the nurse represents both the profession and the health care system and a breakdown in the therapeutic relationship may result in a subsequent lack of trust in a health care service as a whole.

Over to you

Select one complaint that has been made by a patient about nursing in your place of work during the last three months.

What was the complaint about?

Did the complaint indicate a breakdown in the therapeutic relationship? If so, how do you think this happened and why?

- The therapeutic nurse–patient relationship is a relationship that has a defined purpose and duration.
- The kind of person the nurse is has a direct bearing on the type of therapeutic relationships that he or she will form with patients.
- Learning to nurse involves becoming aware of ourselves, our own values and beliefs and how these may affect our relationships with patients.

Caring for patients with long-term conditions

The expression *long-term health conditions* refers to those conditions that present enduring or permanent challenges to an individual's internal environment and to that person's ability to interact with the social or physical world outside the self. These conditions were until recently referred to as *chronic disease/illness*, but current ideas about the nature of health have caused a re-evaluation of this term and recognition that their presence does not define the whole individual. Rather, a long-term health problem is one aspect of who and what a person is. It may have pronounced effects on the way in which that person can live their life but she or he is far more than the asthma, diabetes, haemophilia or hypertension or any other condition from which they suffer. Caring for people with long-term conditions presents many challenges to the primary care nurse.

Case study

Paul Fletcher, aged 35, lives on the edge of a large industrial city and runs a small-holding on which he grows organic vegetables. He also maintains a flock of free-range hens. He has suffered from asthma since infancy. This means that he experiences episodes of bronchospasm that affect his ability to breathe, particularly to exhale. This happens at certain times of the year, particularly during the summer months and early autumn, but it can also occur for other reasons. He has salbutamol via a ventolin accuhaler 200 micrograms, which he uses whenever he feels breathless, but last weekend this did not seem to help.

Saturday was a fine day with a mild breeze blowing from the direction of the city. He stopped digging to have a cigarette after which his chest began to feel tight and his breathing became uncomfortable. He used his inhaler several times during the next forty minutes, but the situation did not improve. The local health centre was closed for the weekend so his wife drove him to the accident and emergency department in the local hospital. On arrival his breathing was rapid and shallow at 28 breaths per minute and pulse oximetry showed an oxygen saturation score of 86 per cent. His pulse rate was 110 beats per minute. His peak flow was unrecordable. He was too breathless to speak more than a few words and had to stop several times when walking from the waiting room to the treatment area. His temperature was normal. He recovered after treatment with salbutamol given via a nebuliser and was eventually discharged home on Sunday with instructions to visit his general practitioner (GP) on Monday morning and to stop smoking. It is now Monday evening. Paul was too busy this morning to make an appointment to see the GP. When his wife arrived home from work she insisted that he visit the health centre. The new practice nurse is an asthma specialist and is free to see him.

Mary Moloney was diagnosed with asthma shortly after she started school. She is now 16 years old and has had frequent hospital admissions with severe bronchospasm. Her family has recently moved into the area and she has come with her mother to register as a patient at the health centre. Mary is very worried about her asthma. She is about to start at the local sixth form college to study for A levels as a first step towards becoming a barrister. The new practice nurse assesses her. She finds that Mary has been using a combination of salbutamol 200 micrograms via ventolin accuhaler as required, beclometasone 200 micrograms via becotide accuhaler twice daily and salmeterol 50 micrograms via serevent accuhaler twice daily. In addition, Mary complains of a stabbing pain in the right lower part of her chest. Coughing aggravates the pain.

What factors should the practice nurse include when assessing these two patients?

How might the practice nurse develop a plan of care that will help both patients to manage their asthma effectively?

What further, long-term strategies are needed?

Sources that will help you learn more about asthma and asthma management: *Nurse Prescribers' Formulary 2003–5.* London, British Medical Association; The National Asthma Campaign at www.asthma.org.uk.

Both patients require a holistic assessment that provides a detailed picture of their circumstances, current health problems and the effects that these may have both now and in the future. This assessment will enable the nurse to construct a total database as a foundation for further action and it will include clarifying Paul and Mary's understanding of asthma, how they feel it affects them and the strategies they use to control it. Listening to patients' accounts of their health problems enables the practice nurse to gain insight into the unique experiences of each patient and helps to make clear how and when problems arise. In addition to listening, the practice nurse will also conduct a physical examination to assess respiratory function and other body systems as well as a review of each patient's technique for using an inhaler. By the end of the assessment the nurse will have collected an extensive amount of information that must then be collated and assessed in the light of professional knowledge to inform the development of a nursing diagnosis and individual asthma management plans (Jarvis 2000; Cohen *et al.* 1998).

In Paul's case the nurse identifies a number of factors in his surroundings to which he may be having an allergic reaction:

feathers from the hens, pollen or spores in the air during the summer and early autumn. Even some of the vegetables he grows may produce such a reaction. Consequently, further investigations will be required and the practice nurse may wish to add an antihistamine to his regular medication. The choice of drug would be influenced by the need to avoid substances that might cause him to feel drowsy if driving or operating machinery. Alongside the possibility of allergy are other factors, some of which are outside Paul's control. For example, although he may live on the edge of a city, quite possibly in a semi-rural area, wind may carry pollution from the city and, in some instances, aggravate his asthma. Paul will not be able to avoid this situation, but he needs to understand the importance of managing his condition to prevent or at least reduce bronchospasm. This may be triggered by occasional exposure to pollution, but in his case it is likely to occur more often as the result of poor management, under-treatment and smoking. If he does not adopt a more proactive approach to asthma, repeated episodes of bronchospasm will cause permanent changes in the air passages of his lungs and in the shape of his chest. These changes cause increasing breathlessness, which will eventually become constant, affecting every aspect of his life.

In Mary's case asthma does not so far seem to be triggered by any identifiable factors, but she too may have allergies that require some investigation. Her frequent admissions to hospital suggest several possibilities that the nurse will need to explore. Mary's current medication may be insufficient for her needs. She and her family may not understand what asthma is or how to use the medication correctly. As an adolescent she may feel self-conscious about using her inhalers or have been the victim of bullying at school because her asthma makes her a little different to the other pupils. She may be suffering from stress as a result of moving to a new area and starting at a new college.

Finally, Mary is complaining of pain in the right side of her chest. As the first point of contact with the health care system, primary care practitioners must avoid making assumptions. For example, the nurse might assume that the pain in Mary's chest is due to her asthma and excessive coughing. It could be so but it might also be indicative of pleurisy, that is, inflammation of the pleura surrounding the lungs, and thus not connected to Mary's asthma at all. Formulating an accurate diagnosis is not as straightforward as it may appear. A patient who presents with chest pain, for example, may have a myocardial infarction, angina or indigestion and it can be difficult, initially, to make a **differential diagnosis**, that is, to differentiate accurately between these possibilities. The causes of

Keywords

Differential diagnosis

Formulating a diagnosis from a collection of signs and symptoms that indicate more than one possibility.

conditions such as multiple sclerosis and anorexia nervosa are uncertain and the symptoms that patients experience may not match formal diagnostic criteria (Seedhouse 1991). Failure to diagnose correctly, or at the very least to recognise that a patient's symptoms warrant further action, increases patient suffering. It can mean that individuals are subjected to inappropriate interventions and that preventable complications develop unchecked. Primary care practitioners are, therefore, responsible for initiating a differential diagnosis and, if necessary, referring the patient to secondary care.

Following assessment the nurse will work with each patient to develop an asthma management plan. Depending on individual need, preferences and lifestyle, this may include adjustments to medication, education about asthma and advice about lifestyle changes to promote better health and education about the correct use of inhalers. The nurse will also ensure that each plan is regularly reviewed to ensure that it is effective. Reviews provide opportunities for physical measurements such as peak flow recordings to be added to the data collected during the initial consultation and thus enable the practitioner to determine whether the patient is showing sufficient sign of improvement or whether further intervention is necessary (Jarvis 2000). Reviews also help the nurse to obtain further insight into each patient's ability and motivation with regard to control of their asthma and clarify those factors that they cannot influence. The aim is to help Paul and Mary incorporate successful asthma management into their lives, cope effectively with episodes of breathlessness and prevent damage to their lungs that will cause long-term respiratory disability.

Key points Top tips

- Primary care practitioners have a major part to play in helping patients with long-term conditions to manage their health problems and improve their quality of life.
- Holistic approaches to the assessment of a patient with a long-term condition enables the primary care nurse to establish that person's attitude to and understanding of their condition as well as their physical state.
- In assessing patients it is important to remember that several conditions have similar signs and symptoms and that the practitioner must make a differential diagnosis.
- Regular reviews are essential in monitoring progress.

Reducing hospital admissions

Hospital admissions will remain a possibility because, even with very good management plans, patients like Paul and Mary are still at risk of sudden exacerbations of their asthma that may be severe or even life threatening. Such episodes may be caused by infection, exposure to allergens and stress. People who suffer from epilepsy, diabetes and some other long-term conditions will have similar episodes of severe illness requiring hospital admission. Such admissions can disrupt the normal management plans and, in the past, communication between primary and secondary care providers has been limited, resulting in disjointed, unsatisfactory care. Recent reforms of the National Health Service are intended to provide better help and care for patients (NHS Modernisation Agency 2004). This is particularly important for older adults who frequently suffer from more than one long-term condition and who therefore may have highly complex care needs (DOH 2005). Nurses working in primary care are to develop new roles as *community matrons*. Community matrons are experienced, skilled nurses who will use case management techniques to help patients who depend on health service support because they have one or more long-term conditions. Such techniques will include drawing together professionals from different disciplines to create care plans based on multi-professional working (a full discussion of multi-professional working is provided in Chapter 8). The aim is to help patients to manage their condition as independently as possible, prevent unnecessary admissions to hospital and, when admissions are essential, reduce the length of their stay. Community matrons will also work to provide better communication between primary and secondary service providers to promote seamless care (DOH 2005). Community matrons will therefore be responsible for identifying and monitoring high-risk patients and, when they are admitted to hospital, instigating an *in-reach programme*. This means that the community matron will work with hospital staff to plan discharge and incorporate recommended changes into the patient's long-term management plan (NHS Modernisation Agency 2004).

Key points Top tips

Multi-professional working in primary care is directed towards promoting independence as far as possible among patients with long-term conditions and reducing hospital admissions.

> **Over to you**
>
> Look up Department of Health (2005) *Supporting People with Long Term Conditions. Liberating the Talents of Nurses Who Care For People With Long Term Conditions.* London, DOH. This can be located at www.dh.gov.uk/publications. Try to answer the following questions:
> - What is case management?
> - How is it envisaged that community matrons will use case management?
> - How many patients will each community matron be responsible for?
> - What is the Evercare model of case management?
> - In your opinion, what are the strengths and weaknesses of this model?

Actively promoting health

Caring for patients with long-term conditions requires primary care nurses to provide education and support that facilitates independence. Working in primary care provides many other opportunities for working with patients to help them improve their knowledge, understanding and skills in relation to health. While many of these opportunities arise in the day-to-day experience of patient care, others are determined by current health policy. One example of the way in which health policy is implemented is through the work of the Healthcare Commission, which is concerned with standards in health care. The Commission inspects and assesses the performance of organisations that provide health care both in the NHS and in the independent sector, in both secondary and primary care settings. The assessment is based around specific targets that each type of organisation is expected to achieve and the standards required.

> **Over to you**
>
> Look up the Healthcare Commission website at www.healthcarecommission.org.uk.
>
> What does the Commission do?
>
> What are the performance indicators for primary care?
>
> Which of the targets set for primary care trusts have implications for patient education?
>
> To locate the information required, look for features in the menu that focus on *service provider information* and/or *NHS performance ratings* for the current year.

Over to you

Look up the following organisations and make brief notes about the role and responsibilities of each one:

- National Institute of Clinical Excellence at www.nice.org.uk;
- NHS Modernisation Agency at www.modern.nhs.uk;
- Strategic Health Authorities at www.nhs.uk/england/authoritiesTrusts/sha/list.aspx – look particularly at the Strategic Health Authority that covers the area in which you live;
- Primary Care Trusts at www.nhs.uk/england/authoritiesTrusts/sha/list.aspx: click on 'Primary Care Trusts' in the left-hand column and then listing in the right-hand column – look particularly at the Primary Care Trust that covers the area in which your GP is located;
- Mental Health Trusts at www.nhs.uk/england/authoritiesTrusts/sha/list.aspx: click on 'Mental Health Trusts' in the left-hand column and then listing in the right-hand column.

In primary care the Healthcare Commission targets and standards can be grouped in terms of broad health issues (see box below). The first group concerns the accessibility and appropriateness of the services provided for the local population. This means that services should be designed to meet the needs of local people and that there should be equity in access, that is to say, that everyone should be able to use services on an equal basis. Where groups of people are socially marginalised, for example those with certain types of mental illness, the development of *assertive outreach* is intended to ensure that they receive the treatments and care required. Teams of practitioners work with mental health service clients, helping those individuals to identify factors that may lead to an exacerbation of their difficulties and to pre-empt the development of crises that may lead to hospitalisation.

Healthcare Commission targets for primary care

1   Ensure that services are appropriate to and accessible by members of the local population
2   Reduce dependence on illicit substances, alcohol and tobacco
3   Prevent illness and disease
4   Improve the management of long-term conditions
5   Ensure the protection of children and young people and reduce teenage pregnancies
6   Obtain feedback from staff about the impact of changes intended to improve their working lives
7   Determine patient satisfaction with the services they use

The second group of Healthcare Commission targets and standards are concerned with dependence on illicit drugs, alcohol and tobacco. For example, smoking is one of the most frequent causes of preventable illness in the UK. The Healthcare Commission aimed to reduce the number of smokers by 800,000 in 2005. However, while people who smoke may wish to give up, the addictive quality of nicotine makes this a difficult and daunting undertaking. The Healthcare Commission has set targets to encourage Primary Care Trusts, and therefore practitioners, to provide structured support programmes to enable smokers to give up tobacco over a period of four weeks.

A third set of Healthcare Commission targets and standards is concerned with the prevention of illness and disease. Regular screening provides one strategy for prevention. For example, cervical screening is estimated to save about 8,000 lives each year. Influenza can be a serious illness in elderly people and in those with certain long-term health conditions such as asthma. Primary care practitioners are therefore expected to ensure that 70 per cent of patients over the age of 65 are offered, and take up, vaccination against influenza and that younger patients at risk are also given the opportunity to prevent this illness.

The fourth group of Healthcare Commission targets and standards concerns improvements in the management of long-term conditions in ways that reduce the possible development of complications, thus saving lives in some instances and improving the quality of life in others. For example, if a patient experiences a heart attack, further damage and complications can be prevented by the administration of *thrombolytic therapy*, which prevents clotting and helps restore an uninterrupted flow of blood through the coronary artery. This therapy is most effective if it is administered within the first hour after the onset of symptoms. Consequently, targets have been set to ensure that patients can derive the maximum benefit from thrombolytic therapy.

The fifth group of Healthcare Commission targets and standards is about the welfare of children and young people through child protection, the prevention of pregnancies among teenage girls and improvements in infant health. This last target is particularly concerned with educating women in socially disadvantaged groups about factors such as the benefits of breastfeeding and the avoidance of smoking during pregnancy.

The last two groups of Healthcare Commission targets and standards focus on the experience of giving and receiving health services. Health service reforms are intended to improve the working lives of staff, for example, through family-friendly employment arrangements and zero tolerance of violence or abuse from service users. Healthcare Commission targets require health service employers to conduct staff surveys to determine the extent and impact of such improvements. Alongside the experiences of staff are concerns about service users and their satisfaction with the services provided. Thus Healthcare Commission targets also require Trusts to undertake patient satisfaction surveys and, if necessary, find other ways of ascertaining patients' views.

Inherent in each of the Healthcare Commission targets and standards is the need for education for:

- patients and their families to help them improve their health;
- practitioners to enable them to find new ways of working.

Providing this education involves far more than simply delivering information that people may not understand or regard as relevant to them. Even if they understand the information, some patients or practitioners may not know how to incorporate the information into their lifestyles or working practices. Others may find the process of changing so difficult that they give up. Information must, therefore, be accompanied by guidance and coaching that empowers an individual to work through a **transition,** that is, 'a passage from one life phase, condition or status . . . to another' (Chick and Meleis 1986 pp. 239–40).

Coaching and guiding patients, families or colleagues through transitions begin with the identification of the type of transition to be made (Spross *et al.* 2000):

- A *developmental transition* is one that relates to the lifecycle. For example, coaching women to give up smoking during pregnancy and learn how to breastfeed would be part of helping them make the transition into parenthood.
- A *health–illness transition* is one that is directly related to helping people manage their own health. It might, for example, include helping a patient to make suitable lifestyle adjustments following a heart attack or enabling older adults to appreciate the risks of influenza and take the opportunity to prevent it.
- An *organisational transition* is one in which an organisation as a whole goes through a period of change. Current health service reforms require NHS Trusts to introduce a wide range of changes to improve the quality of services and the experiences of patients who use them (DOH 1997). Enabling a Trust to develop outreach teams or make existing services more accessible are two examples of this type of transition, although it could also be argued that the entire health service is in a state of organisational transition.

⚷ *Keywords*

Transition

A period of change during which the individual adjusts from one set of circumstances to another.

- A *situational transition* is one in which changes in role or the workplace setting are required. Gee (1998) described a situational transition in which she provided coaching and guiding for a team of nursing staff to enable them to administer thrombolytic therapy to patients following a heart attack. At first the nurses were reluctant and resistant to taking on new responsibilities. However, as an expert in cardiology nursing, Gee was able to work with them in clinical practice and identify the likely impact of these responsibilities on their roles and workload. She was then able to devise a strategy for change that took account of the nurses' concerns, and provided practical demonstrations and the opportunity to practise, alongside an expert, within informal workshops. Thus nurses felt supported in learning new skills and incorporating these into their regular practice (Gee 1998).

Reflective activity

Select two patients whom you have nursed recently.

Identify the types of transitions they were making.

What knowledge and skills would you need to help them make these transitions?

Gee's (1998) account indicates that providing coaching and guidance requires a high level of clinical knowledge and technical skills to be able to show others what is required and enable them to become competent and confident practitioners or managers of their own health. Alongside these skills the nurse must have the ability to relate to people, to find out how they view a particular situation and work with them in bringing about change (Spross *et al.* 2000). Thus coaching and guiding requires interpersonal competence, and the ability to communicate with others effectively and build therapeutic nurse-patient relationships with patients or families and sound working relationships with colleagues. Both these relationships require a caring, sensitive approach to others based on an understanding of the nature of the transition required, the context in which it is to take place and the ability to creatively apply professionals skills.

Furthermore, the nurse must recognise that transitions do not occur in isolation. A woman who requires coaching and guiding through the developmental transition of pregnancy may also need help in making a health–illness transition if she experiences complications or has to adapt the management of a long-term condition to protect her baby. Both these transitions may take place while she is using services that are in the process of organisational transition or in which the staff are making the situational transitions required in learning new ways of working. This means that the provision of education in terms of providing information and empowering people to use it is a complex activity in which the nurse may have to contend with several competing priorities at the same time.

Key points | Top tips

- The Healthcare Commission sets targets and standards for Primary Care Trusts about a range of issues to do with service provision.
- These targets require primary care practitioners to educate patients more effectively.
- Practitioners themselves require education to help them develop new ways of working.

Conclusion

This chapter has helped you to examine critically the concept of health in relation to the nursing metaparadigm and within the context of primary health care. Nursing roles in primary care provide opportunities to bring about health improvements by working with patients and families, empowering them to use information to bring about changes in their lifestyles or in the management of long-term conditions.

RRRRRRapid recap

1   What is the main focus of primary care?
2   How do long-term health conditions affect patients?
3   What is the role of community matrons?
4   What is the role of the Healthcare Commission?

References

Campinha-Bacote, J. (2003) *The Process of Cultural Competence in the Delivery of Healthcare Services: A Culturally Competent Model of Care,* 4th edition. Available from Transcultural Care Associates at www.transculturalcare.net.

Chick and Meleis, A. (1986) 'Transitions: a nursing concern', in P. Chinn (ed.) *Nursing Research Methodology: Issues and Implementation*, Rockville MD, Aspen Publishers, pp. 237–58.

Close, A. (2003) 'Advanced practice and health promotion', Chapter 10 in P. McGee and G. Castledine (eds) *Advanced Practice*, 2nd edn. Oxford, Blackwell Science, pp. 112–28.

Cohen, S., Bailey, P. P., Begemann, C. and Moffett, K. (1998) 'Advanced physical assessment', Chapter 6 in G. Castledine and P. McGee (eds) *Advanced and Specialist Nursing Practice*. Oxford, Blackwell Science, pp. 93–118.

Department of Health (DOH) (1997) *The New NHS. Modern, Dependable*. London, DOH.

Department of Health (DOH) (2004) *The NHS Improvement Plan: Putting People at the Heart of Public Services,* London, DOH.

Department of Health (DOH) (2005) *Supporting People with Long Term Conditions: Liberating the Talents of Nurses who Care for People with Long Term Conditions,* London, DOH.

Fawcett, J. (2000) *Analysis and Evaluation of Contemporary Nursing Knowledge: Nursing Models and Theories*, 2nd edn. Philadellphia PA, F. A. Davis.

Gee, K. (1998) 'The roles of consultant and researcher in advanced cardiology nursing', Chapter 16 in G. Castledine and P. McGee (eds) *Advanced and Specialist Practice*. Oxford, Blackwell Science, pp. 192–8.

Howk, C. (2002) 'Hildegard E. Peplau: psychodynamic nursing', Chapter 21 in A. Marriner Tomey and R. A. Alligood (eds) *Nursing Theorists and Their Work,* 5th edn. St Louis MO, C. V. Mosby, pp. 379–98.

Jarvis, C. (2000) *Physical Examination and Health Assessment,* 3rd edn. Philadelphia PA, W. B. Saunders.

King, I. (1981) *A Theory for Nursing: Systems, Concepts, Process*. New York, John Wiley and Sons.

Neuman, B. and Fawcett, J. (2002) *The Neuman Systems Model*. Upper Saddle River NJ, Prentice Hall.

NHS Modernisation Agency (2004) *Chronic Disease Management. Unique Care*. Available at www.natpact.nhs.uk/cms/403.php.

Nightingale, F. (1860/1969) *Notes on Nursing: What It Is and What It Is Not*. New York, Dover Publications.

Peplau, H. (1952) *Interpersonal Relations in Nursing*. New York, G. P. Putnam.

Seedhouse, D. (1991) *Liberating Medicine*. Chichester, John Wiley and Sons.

Simpson, H. (1991) *Peplau's Model in Action*. Basingstoke, Macmillan.

Spross, J., Clarke, E. and Beauregard, J. (2000) 'Expert coaching and guidance', Chapter 7 in A. Hamric, J. Spross and C. Hanson (eds) *Advanced Nursing Practice. An Integrative Approach*, 3rd edn. Philadelphia PA, W. B. Saunders, pp. 183–210.

World Health Organization (1946) Constitution. Geneva, WHO.

6

Culture and care

Learning outcomes

By the end of this chapter you should be able to:

- briefly explain the concept of culture and why it is important in health care;

- demonstrate an understanding of some of the common cultural issues that may arise in caring for patients;

- briefly explain the concept of cultural competence and discuss one approach to using this to provide care for patients.

Introduction

Culture is a learned way of thinking and feeling that is shared with others and that provides a particular way of being in and experiencing the world. It is a type of 'mental software' (Hofstede 1994). Culture is, therefore, an attribute of every individual, just as software programs are an integral part of every computer. Culture is first encountered in the home, where parents, grandparents and other family members socialise children into a particular way of life based on specific beliefs, values, customs and traditions that can briefly be summed up as 'the way we live our lives'. Later on, children encounter the cultures of their schools and colleges in which they are taught 'how we do things around here' as opposed to establishments elsewhere. In adult life, each place of work, each group of work colleagues, each profession, each group of friends has a set of values, beliefs, customs and traditions that influence the ways in which they function. An individual may, therefore, belong to several different cultures at the same time – that of home, work, friends, team mates – and have to adapt to each one. This is a part of normal everyday life and, like culture itself, it is taken for granted. We do not think consciously about the cultures to which we belong or how we should behave in any of them. Indeed, if anyone asked 'What is your culture?', you would probably find it very difficult to describe, because there are individual preferences and differences in addition to the taken-for-granted element. Even if it is possible to describe a culture, there will still be more variation between individual members of that culture than between it and others (Helman 2000).

Culture and cultural diversity are, therefore, features of everyday life. It is only when individuals encounter values, customs, beliefs and traditions that seem quite different that they become aware of their own. Having to think consciously about things we normally take for granted can feel strange and uncomfortable. It also presents us with challenges about how we need to adapt to fit in with a new situation. This chapter helps you to consider the ways in which cultural differences can present challenges for the nurse and to develop appropriate strategies that will help you to provide care in circumstances in which you and your patient do not share the same cultural heritage. The chapter begins with a discussion of the reasons why culture is important in health care. It helps you to identify the ways in which cultural issues can arise in the process of providing care and enables you to develop an understanding of one approach to providing culturally appropriate care.

The importance of culture in health care

If culture is a way of being in and experiencing the world, then it is logical to assume that it will affect our views and ideas about health and illness. What we think makes us healthy or ill, how illness should be treated and how the sick should be cared for are all determined by our cultural values, beliefs, customs and traditions.

Reflective activity

Think about the last time you were ill:
- What do you think caused that illness and why?
- How would you describe that illness?
- Who did you tell about your illness?
- What did you expect that person to do?
- If you went to see a doctor, what happened?
- Was this what you expected?

Health, illness, treatment and care are universal phenomena, but each culture provides a unique explanation of why people become sick and how health may be regained (Leininger and McFarland 2002). Professional nursing socialises students into thinking that illness is the result of biological or psychological challenges with which the individual cannot cope, but for many people, cultural values and beliefs provide quite different explanations in which illness is regarded as the result of a breakdown in relationships between people or between them and the supernatural. For example, an individual might say 'I have cancer because I didn't make things up with my mother before she died.' Alternatively, illness may be conceptualised as disharmony within the self or between the self and the external social or physical world (Helman 2000). Professionals who arbitrarily dismiss such beliefs not only run the risk of giving offence but also undermine their own attempts to provide treatment and care that patients feel they can trust, and that is congruent with what they consider appropriate. To be effective, care must be perceived by the patient as relevant and meaningful in nature and in the manner in which it is delivered (Leininger and McFarland 2002).

Every culture has systems in place to care for the sick. These may take the form of traditional healing practices, complementary therapists or formal systems of medicine. Traditional healing practices are those based on knowledge, skill and tradition within a specific culture. Those who carry out such practices do not have formal, professional training but are, nevertheless, trusted by members of a culturally based community to provide help in ways that are consistent with their values and beliefs (Nolan 1989). Alongside traditional healers, there exists a wide range of other practitioners, such as osteopaths, therapeutic massage practitioners, homeopaths and chiropractors, who undergo formal training. They function outside, but in a complementary manner to, the established health services. Formal systems of medicine form a third system. One example is that of Chinese medicine, which is now widely available in the UK. This is based on ideas about health as a state of harmony and balance between two different forces, Yin and Yang (Chen 2001). These ideas provide a basis for a holistic approach to care that extends beyond physical treatment into both social relationships and the environment. For example, all illness is classified in terms of either Yin or Yang. Medication is also classified in the same way. A patient with a Yin illness, such as cancer, must be treated with Yang medication in order to restore harmony and health (Estes 1998; Andrews and Boyle 2003).

Reflective activity

Patients may access help from several different sources – traditional healing practices, complementary therapists, or formal, non-Western systems of medicine What do you think are the possible implications of this for nursing practice?

Whatever their cultural beliefs and practices regarding health, patients are entitled to respect. Recent developments in thinking about human rights have highlighted the issue of cultural diversity and contributed to changes in UK legislation that aim to protect individuals from discrimination based on perceived differences (Charter of Fundamental Rights of the European Union 2000, European Convention on Human Rights, Human Rights Act 1998, Race Relations (Amendment) Act 2002). Alongside these legal changes, current health policy is intended to increase the accessibility and availability of services, particularly for those who are socially marginalised because, for example, their values and beliefs are at odds with those of the dominant majority of the population (DOH 1997, 2000). Professional bodies have also been influenced by ideas about human rights, and nurses working in the UK are now required to comply with a code of professional conduct in which they are charged with responsibility to promote and protect the interests and dignity of patients, irrespective of gender, age, race, ability, sexuality, economic status, lifestyle, culture and religious or political beliefs (NMC 2002). These legal, policy and professional changes have served to place cultural diversity at the centre of nursing as one of the key considerations in the provision of good quality care for patients.

Key points | Top tips

- Culture is an aspect of every individual and helps to provide a framework or blueprint for a way of living.
- Culture is taken for granted until we meet someone whose cultural values and beliefs are different to our own.
- Culture is important in health care because:
  - it influences what people think about health and illness and their views about care;
  - nurses have a professional responsibility to show respect for cultural values and beliefs and to ensure that everyone receives appropriate care;
  - current health service reforms aim to widen access to care, making services more appropriate to the cultural and other needs of local populations.

Cultural issues in care

Cultural diversity has implications for the ways in which nurses assess patients, identify their problems, formulate diagnoses and deliver care. There are two ways of approaching this:

- existing assessment frameworks can be expanded to incorporate cultural issues;

- specific assessments tools can be used alongside those assessment frameworks.

Theory into Practice

Identify the advantages and disadvantages of expanding the assessment framework that you use in practice.

What aspects of that framework would have to be developed and why?

Expanding existing frameworks for nursing assessment

Some nursing theories allow the nurse to incorporate cultural issues into the collection of other information about the patient. For example, Roper *et al.* (2000) state that the activities of living are influenced by sociocultural factors and may include cultural diversity. Consideration of each activity – for example, eating and drinking, communication and dying – clearly raises questions about cultural values and beliefs. However, the authors have not addressed these is any detail, and consequently the nurse may find it difficult to determine which questions to ask or how to interpret the answers (see Table 6.1).

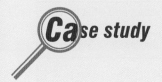
Case study

Balbinder Kaur Gill, aged 35 years, lives with her husband and their three young children. The couple run a supermarket, which requires them to work very long hours, getting up at 5 a.m. to receive the newspapers and other deliveries. The shop is open every day, from 6 a.m. until 7.30 p.m., except Sunday. Balbinder is always busy and tired.

Five years ago she suddenly began to lose weight and felt thirsty all the time. Tests showed that she had diabetes and she was prescribed insulin. Since then, Balbinder has been admitted several times to hospital as an emergency with hypoglycaemia (low blood sugar). Balbinder speaks good English and has assured staff in the local health centre and at the hospital that she is taking her insulin regularly and following the dietary advice she has been given. Staff in both places feel exasperated with her and think that she is not telling the truth.

In May Balbinder went home to India to visit her relations, who live in a country village. While she was there, her diabetes seemed to go away and she did not feel that she still needed treatment so she stopped taking her insulin. When she came back to England in the middle of August she felt very well, but now the thirst and weight loss have started again and she has been admitted to hospital.

In what ways might cultural factors be influencing this situation?

Table 6.1 Sociocultural factors that affect the activities of living	
Activities of living	**Sociocultural factors that affect each activity**
Maintaining a safe environment	Safety and what is deemed responsible behaviour are culturally determined because each setting and each part of the world generates specific hazards.
Communication	Language, local dialect, non-verbal signs and religion.
Breathing	Smoking and spitting.
Eating and drinking	The foods that people eat; the ways in which they both prepare and eat it.
Eliminating	Authors have little to say about sociocultural factors affecting this activity.
Personal cleansing and dressing	Ideas about personal hygiene and dress.
Controlling body temperature	Social norms regarding behaviour in hot and cold environments.
Mobilising	Certain factors, including religion, may influence the type of sporting activities and other forms of exercise in which individuals engage.
Working and playing	Gender and religion, but authors give little information about this.
Expressing sexuality	Religion and gender impinge on sexual behaviour, which is discussed with particular reference to permissiveness in Western society and the spread of AIDS.
Sleeping	Where a person sleeps, with whom and what they wear.
Dying	Social and religious customs surrounding death.

Source: Summarised from Roper *et al.* (2000)

The patient's name will be among the first items of information that the nurse collects in any assessment. Names convey a considerable amount of information about an individual. For example, Western naming systems convey information about gender, family, age, fashion and, in the case of women, marital status. Convention requires that the names be presented in a specific order so that it is clear which is the family name. However some first names can be used for both genders and some names can be used either as first or family names.

> ## Over to you
>
> Write down your full name.
>
> What information does this convey to others about you?
>
> Is there a form of your name that only your family/close friends use?
>
> Is there a form of your name that you consider formal? When do you expect this to be used?
>
> When you meet someone for the first time, do you:
>
> - smile and shake hands?
> - smile but not shake hands?
> - bow with your hands pressed together in front of you?
>
> Give reasons for your actions.

Balbinder's name indicates that she is a Sikh woman. Sikh names have three components. The first/personal name does not indicate gender. The last name is the family name. The middle name indicates both gender and religion: kaur (princess) = woman; singh (lion-hearted) = man. Sikhism emphasises equality: thus all men are equal as are all women. There are no distinctions to be made between the genders and no titles or castes, although some families may interpret the religious teaching in different ways. Understanding this emphasis on equality challenges prevailing stereotypes about South Asian people, particularly those concerning women.

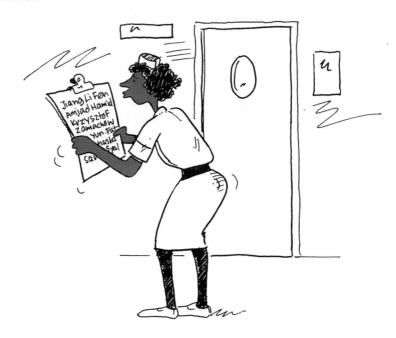

The patient's medical diagnosis is relevant to the nursing assessment as it may influence the type of care required and the way in which it is provided. Balbinder has diabetes, a condition that is increasingly common, particularly among people of South Asian origin (www.diabetesuffolk.com). Reasons for this are unclear but they are thought to relate to dietary changes, increases in obesity and lack of exercise, although there is no indication that any of these apply to her. Management of her condition requires the administration of regular injections of insulin to enable her body to utilise glucose at cellular level. Unless insulin is present, glucose cannot enter cells to provide energy and so remains in the bloodstream. High levels of blood glucose cause damage to blood vessels and the organs they serve, leading to long-term and permanent damage to eyes, kidneys, heart, brain and circulatory systems. Patient education plays a vital part in reducing these complications. It is possible that Balbinder has not really understood or received sufficient teaching about the management of her diabetes. This in itself is not a cultural issue but her underlying beliefs about the nature and causation of illness may have a bearing on her situation. When she went to India on holiday she probably did not have to get up so early in the morning or work very long days. She was, no doubt, able to relax and enjoy herself and consequently felt less tired. She probably walked everywhere and thus had more exercise. Consequently, some of the troubling signs of her diabetes may have receded, leading her to believe that it had gone away. She might also have used some traditional remedies that, like insulin, served to lower blood glucose levels. Thus nursing assessment should include some questions about Balbinder's holiday, not to blame or criticise her but to develop a clearer understanding of her learning needs with regard to the management of her condition.

Effective education begins with and builds on the patient's knowledge of her condition, but professionals also have to consider whether the teaching that they provide is culturally appropriate. Too often professionals give advice and education that is *ethnocentric*, that is, rooted in their own values, beliefs and traditions. They then expect patients to comply, without considering individuals' cultures or lifestyles. Balbinder may have been instructed to take her insulin at times that are inappropriate, given the hours that she has to work in the shop, and do not fit in with her lifestyle. Similarly the timing of meals in a South Asian household is not the same as in other cultures. For instance, the evening meal may not be taken until quite late, about 8 or 9 p.m. If Balbinder has been instructed to take her insulin at 6 p.m., and is complying with that instruction, then it is not surprising that she is having episodes of hypoglycaemia. Current health service reforms have shifted away from notions of

◦━┓ *Keywords*

Compliance

Instructing the patient in what to do without consideration of individual differences or preferences.

Concordance

Negotiating with the patient about the nature and suitability of the care and treatment available to establish a mutually agreed plan of action based on the individual's circumstances.

compliance towards negotiation with the patient, offering choice and discussing with each individual what is appropriate for them. Patient and professional meet on a more equal basis to establish **concordance**. This is an individualised plan to ensure the appropriateness and efficacy of treatment and care (DOH 2003).

Further questioning in the nursing assessment will highlight other activities in which culture may be influential, particularly eating and drinking. As a person who has diabetes Balbinder needs to eat a healthy, balanced diet in which the intake of foods containing carbohydrates, especially those that are processed or refined, is monitored to ensure that blood sugar levels remain stable. Part of the nursing assessment should include consideration of the type of food that Balbinder normally eats and when she eats it as well as her preferences while in hospital.

Assessing cultural issues separately

As an alternative to expanding the existing framework, the nurse could use a separate, cultural assessment tool. A number of nurse theorists argue that this is a better approach because it enables the nurse to undertake a more detailed assessment, contextualise the patient's problems more accurately, and plan and implement appropriate interventions (Leininger and McFarland 2002; Andrews and Boyle 2003; Campinha-Bacote 2003). Separate cultural assessments are described as an essential part of patient care because they encourage a more holistic view of the individual than the traditional physiological or mental health assessments and enable practitioners to develop a positive understanding of culturally based behaviours (Morris 1996). The problem with most of these tools is that they are very detailed and not suited for use in busy health care settings where time is limited. However, there are a few examples of short, practical guides for cultural assessment that help nurses to think more deeply about cultural issues in care. These can be used either as separate assessment tools or to inform the more general assessment framework. One example of a short cultural assessment tool (Naraynan 1997) identifies seven categories that the nurse should consider in relation to cultural issues in care (see next page).

Use of these categories in assessing Balbinder could help the nurse to clarify a number of issues. Attention to *etiquette and social customs* would enable the nurse to understand more about Balbinder's everyday life, such as social mores, how people address and relate to each other, the influence of religion in their lives, and traditions and values pertinent to the management of her diabetes. Finding out about *non-verbal patterns of communication* might help the nurse to understand how these are influenced by culture, i.e. what is considered polite or offensive in both verbal and non-verbal

---

Naraynan's categories for cultural assessment

1 etiquette and social customs
2 non-verbal patterns of communication
3 client's explanation of the problems
4 nutrition
5 pain
6 medication
7 psychosocial factors

Source: Summarised from Naraynan 1997

---

terms. Balbinder's *explanation of her health problems* would provide evidence of her understanding of diabetes and the management of her condition and the ways in which she feels she either copes well or needs help. This information will also help the nurse to clarify Balbinder's views about what will help her most in managing her condition. Care is a universal phenomenon, but members of each culture have particular ideas about what constitutes appropriate care and what does not (Leininger and McFarland 2002). For example, in Western cultures, if a family member other than one's immediate relatives is unwell, it may be sufficient to send a 'get well' card and some flowers. People tend to stay away to leave the individual time to recover. In cultures that originate in countries without a welfare state, this would be considered very uncaring, because it is the family's responsibility to provide care for members who are ill. People demonstrate care by visiting rather than by staying away.

Assessment of Balbinder's *nutrition* would help the nurse to gain a clearer picture of her food intake in relation to her lifestyle. The long hours worked in the shop may make it difficult to prepare family meals or to eat regularly. Consequently she may be relying on snacks to help control her blood sugar levels. *Pain* is a universal phenomenon, but reactions to pain are culturally determined. Modern Western ideas about pain are based on Descartes' division of mind and body. Pain is regarded as a symptom of malfunction requiring the services of a professional who will measure, control and kill it (Illych 1975). However, members of cultures that regard pain as an inescapable part of daily life ascribe responsibility and autonomy to the individual to deal with their own suffering, supported by culturally based rituals and values such as patience and courage. Assessing pain in a patient from a different culture depends on the individual's willingness and ability to talk about it and make the pain a public rather than a private matter. It also depends on the nurse's ability to understand the significance of what is communicated and to accept the possibility of different experiences of and attitudes towards pain.

Over to you

Read Helman, C. (2000) 'Pain and culture', Chapter 7 in C. Helman *Culture Health and Illness*. Oxford, Butterworth Heinemann.

In what ways does culture influence the experience and expression of pain?

What do you regard as acceptable ways of making pain public and why?

What might be the negative consequences of making pain public?

Assessing *medication* would help the nurse to clarify Balbinder's understanding of her insulin and her technique when injecting herself. The timing of her insulin doses and the effectiveness of her blood sugar monitoring coupled with information about her lifestyle would provide a useful basis for establishing concordance. Finally, attention to *psychosocial factors* might help the nurse to establish how Balbinder feels about her diabetes, how it affects her life and some of the pressures she may be experiencing both psychologically and socially (Kinmond *et al.* 2003).

Thus, in using this separate cultural assessment tool, the nurse may be able to develop a more detailed picture of the patient's circumstances as a basis for planning and delivering culturally appropriate care. It may prove useful when assessing patients with long-term conditions or complex health care needs. However, the introduction of a separate assessment tool may militate against its use. Staff may simply forget it or regard it as yet another piece of paper to fill in rather than something that will help them. Regardless of the approach selected – expanding the existing framework or introducing a separate cultural assessment – success depends on the nurse's

- ability to recognise the impact that cultural factors may have on the experience of health and illness and the motivation to address these factors in the provision of care;
- knowledge and experience of cultural diversity to interpret correctly the information provided and utilise it appropriately.

Assumptions and simple intuitive reactions to the information that patients present are not valid and can lead to misdiagnosis and inappropriate treatment (Paniagua 1998; Tuck 1984). In other words, nurses need to become culturally competent.

- Care is a universal phenomenon but each culture provides specific ideas about how care should be given.
- Cultural ideas about care have implications for the way in which nurses assess patients through:
  - adapting existing assessment frameworks;
  - using separate assessment tools.
- Practitioners need to move beyond cultural stereotypes and ethnocentric thinking towards culturally competent practice.
- Negotiating concordance rather than compliance is more likely to help patients to manage their health problems in culturally appropriate ways.

Providing culturally competent care

The term *cultural competence* refers to the ability of an individual to work effectively within the cultural context of another person. It is also used to describe an organisation's capability in accommodating the cultural values, beliefs and customs of its clients. Becoming culturally competent is a gradual process through which the individual evolves by learning, reflecting and acting (see Figure 6.1). The key elements of cultural competence are: first, respect for, and valuing of, difference and thus recognition of the need to address the inequalities and power relationships that may adversely affect the provision and experience of services; and, second, the requirement that professionals translate that respect and recognition into knowledge and understanding that is applied in their practice in order to improve the quality of care (Betancourt *et al.* 2002 p. 3). These first two elements concern the individual practitioner. A third element concerns the organisations in which practitioners are employed. At organisational level cultural competence requires an organisation to:

- have a defined set of values and principles and demonstrate behaviours, attitudes, policies and structures that enable them to work effectively, i.e. systemic competence (Betancourt *et al.* 2002);
- have the capacity to value diversity, conduct self-assessment, manage the dynamics of difference, acquire and institutionalise cultural knowledge and adapt to diversity and the cultural context of the communities they serve;
- incorporate the above into all aspects of policy making, finance and administration, practice and service delivery, and involve

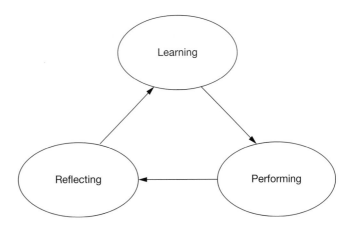

Figure 6.1 *What is cultural competence?*

systematically consumers, key stakeholders and communities
(National Center for Cultural Competence at gucchd.georget
own.edu/nccc/);

- have a capacity to communicate effectively with members of
  diverse groups who may not share the same language,
  communication style and level of literacy or who have other
  characteristics that influence interaction;
- recognise that cultural competence benefits both clients and the
  organisation as a whole.

For cultural competence to become a reality, practitioners and their
employing organisations need to work together to develop
appropriate, good quality care and services (McGee 2000).

The first step in becoming culturally competent is to determine
what is to be achieved and who will benefit. This requires the
initiation of a local *database* to which information can be added over
time. The 2001 census data can provide some useful information
about cultural diversity in the locality, but practitioners require data
that are relevant to their particular services. The census data will
show the broad mix of the local population. Ethnic monitoring
within the health service will provide further data about the
members of diverse cultures who are using particular services and
perhaps indicate sections of the population who should be, but are
not, doing so.

Practitioners then have to consider what they currently know
about local cultural groups, how this information has been gathered
and whether it is accurate. Forming relationships with local people
and consulting with them about what they most value in health
services will gradually add to the initial database.

> ## Over to you
>
> Visit the National Statistics website at
> www.statistics.gov.uk/census2001 for information about the 2001 census:
>
> 1 Roughly what percentage of the population of England and Wales belongs to black or other minority ethnic groups?
> 2 Which are the largest minority ethnic groups in England and Wales?
>
> Click on 'Neighbourhood' at the top of the page and then insert the name of the city/town/place in which you work:
>
> 3 Roughly what percentage of people in that city/town/place belong to black or other minority ethnic groups?
> 4 Which are the largest minority ethnic groups?
> 5 Roughly what percentage of people are under 18 years of age?
> 6 Roughly what percentage of people are over 75 year of age?
>
> Click on 'Back' and insert the name of a local ward:
>
> 7 Roughly what percentage of people in that ward belong to black or minority ethnic groups?
> 8 Which are the largest minority ethnic groups in that ward?
> 9 Roughly what percentage of people is under 18 years of age?
> 10 Roughly what percentage of people is over 75 years of age? Repeat this exercise comparing four different electoral wards in the city or town.
> 11 What do the census data reveal about diversity in your locality?
> 12 In your opinion do the data give you an accurate and complete picture?
> 13 What other information might be useful and where might it be found?

> ## Over to you
>
> Visit the Clinical Governance Support Team site at
> www.cgsupport.nhs.uk. Click on 'Patient Experience'. Make notes about the guidance given on involving patients in any aspect of service provision.
>
> Visit or contact the Patient Advocacy and Liaison Service in your place of work. What is the role and function of this service?

The experience of caring for patients presents many opportunities for nurses to learn about cultural issues and to find ways of *adapting their practice*. Individual practitioners and teams of nurses need to explore ways in which that learning can be shared and incorporated into their repertoire of knowledge and skill (Benner *et al.* 1996; McGee 2000; Campinha-Bacote 2003). Table 6.2 presents a summary of the ways in which skills can be adapted based on cultural knowledge.

Table 6.2 Adapting nursing skills for culturally competent care

Transcultural nursing theory

Transcultural nursing theory provides three options:

1 *Culture care preservation/maintenance:* means working within the patient's frame of reference, for example when teaching parents about weaning, preserving and maintaining cultural values and beliefs.

2 *Culture care accommodation/negotiation:* means helping people to adapt their health practices in order to improve their health in culturally appropriate ways, for example helping people to use traditional remedies safely.

3 *Culture care re-patterning/restructuring:* means helping people cope with imposed changes in culturally appropriate ways, for example managing a stoma.

Source: Leininger and McFarland (2002).

Cultural safety nursing theory

Cultural safety nursing theory provides an additional strategy by asking the nurse to think about the ways in which power is present in the nurse–patient relationship. The practitioner has a position of power with regard to the patient. Cultural safety emphasises the empowerment of the patient. Cultural safety requires professionals to:

1 examine personal values and attitudes;

2 be open-minded and flexible in their approach to people who differ from themselves;

3 avoid blaming the victims of oppression for their condition.

Source: Papps and Ramsden (1996).

The acquisition of knowledge and ability to adapt practice-based skills are both dependent on a third factor, that of the nurse's *self-awareness* and ability to interact constructively. The development of cultural competence requires a deliberate, conscious process of examining the self in ways that enable nurses to become sensitive to the concepts of cultural differences and prejudice within their own lives. Negative attitudes and prejudices will affect their interactions with people from other cultures and adversely affect the therapeutic nurse–patient relationship. What are needed are practitioners who 'strive toward a culturally-liberated interacting style' in which differences are seen positively as part of 'a shared learning experience' with the patient (Campinha-Bacote 1994 p. 9). The object is to become culturally responsive by 'incorporating the individual's beliefs, lifeways and practices into a mutually acceptable treatment plan' (Campinha-Bacote 1994 p. 11). Motivation is a key element of this developing self-awareness, because without this there is no true commitment to change (Campinha-Bacote 2003).

Key points Top tips

- Cultural competence is a continuous process of learning, reflecting and acting in ways that incorporate cultural issues into care.
- Cultural competence is a matter for all practitioners requiring them to:
  - develop a local knowledge database;
  - adapt their practice to meet local need.
- Culturally competent organisations are those that value diversity and seek to incorporate it into every aspect of their work.

Conclusion

This chapter has helped you to examine the impact of culture on the provision of nursing care within the context of a multicultural society. Cultural beliefs and values determine how people conceptualise health and illness, how illness should be treated and what they believe will restore their health. Nurses need to learn about the cultures represented among their patient groups and become competent in providing care for patients of diverse backgrounds.

RRRRRRapid recap

1 Why is culture important in health care?
2 What are the advantages and disadvantages of using existing nursing tools to assess cultural issues in nursing care?
3 What are the advantages and disadvantages of using specific tools to assess cultural issues in nursing care?
4 What is cultural competence?
5 What is concordance?

References

Andrews, M. and Boyle, J. (2003) *Transcultural Concepts in Nursing Care*, 4th edn. London, Lippincott, Williams and Wilkins.

Benner, P., Tanner, C. and Chesla, C. (1996) *Expertise in Nursing Practice. Caring, Clinical Judgement and Ethics*. New York, Springer Publishing Company.

Betancourt, J. R., Green, A. and Carillo, J. E. (2002) *Cultural Competence in Healthcare: Emerging Frameworks and Practical Approaches*. A field report available from the Commonwealth Fund at www.cmwf.org.

Campinha-Bacote, J. (1994) *The Process of Competence in Health Care: A Culturally Competent Model of Health Care*, 2nd edn. Cincinnati OH, Transcultural Care Associates.

Campinha-Bacote, J. (2003) *The Process of Cultural Competence in the Delivery of Healthcare Services: A Culturally Competent Model of Care,* 4th edn. Available from Transcultural Care Associates at www.transculturalcare.net.

Chen, Y. (2001) 'Chinese values, health and nursing', *Journal of Advanced Nursing* 36 (2) pp. 270–3.

Department of Health (DOH) (1997) *The New NHS. Modern, Dependable.* London, DOH.

Department of Health (DOH) (2000) *The NHS Plan. A Plan for Investment. A Plan for Reform.* London, DOH.

Department of Health (DOH) (2003) *Choice, Responsiveness and Equity in the NHS and Social Care. A National Consultation.* London, DOH.

Estes, M. E. Z. (1998) *Health Assessment and Physical Examination.* New York, Delmar Publishers.

Helman, C. (2000) *Culture, Health and Illness.* 4th edn. Oxford, Butterworth Heinemann.

Hofstede, G. (1994) *Culture and Organisations: Software of the Mind. Intercultural Cooperation and its Importance for Survival.* London, HarperCollins.

Illych, I. (1975) *Limits to Medicine: Medical Nemesis – The Expropriation of Health.* London, Marion Boyars Publishers.

Kinmond, K., McGee, P., Gough, S. and Ashford, A. (2003) '"Loss of self": a psychosocial study of the quality of life of adults with diabetic foot ulceration', *Journal of Tissue Viability* 13 (1) pp. 6, 8, 10, 12, 14, 16.

Leininger, M. and McFarland, M. (2002*) Transcultural Nursing: Concepts, Theories, Research and Practice,* 3rd edn. New York, McGraw Hill.

McGee, P. (2000) *Culturally-sensitive Nursing: A Critique.* Unpublished PhD Thesis, Birmingham, University of Central England.

Morris, R. (1996) 'Bridging cultural boundaries: the African American and transcultural caring', *Advanced Practice Nursing Quarterly* 2 (2) pp. 31–8.

Naraynan, M. C. (1997) 'Cultural assessment in home health care', *Home Health Care Nurse* 15 (10) pp. 663–72.

Nolan, P. (1989) 'Folk medicine in rural Ireland', *Journal of Ethnological Stud*ies 27 pp. 44–56.

Nursing and Midwifery Council (NMC) (2002) *Code of Professional Conduct.* London, NMC.

Paniagua, F. (1998) *Assessing and Treating Culturally Diverse Clients. A Practical Guide*, 2nd edn. London, Sage.

Papps, E. and Ramsden, I. (1996) 'Cultural safety in nursing: the New Zealand experience', *International Journal of Quality in Health Care* 8 (5) pp. 491–3.

Roper, N., Logan, W. and Tierney, A. (2000) *The Roper-Logan-Tierney Model of Nursing: Based on Activities of Living.* Edinburgh, Churchill Livingstone.

Tuck, I. (1984) 'Strategies for integrating African American culture in the curriculum', *Journal of Nursing Education* 23 (6) pp. 261–2.

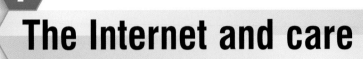

7

The Internet and care

Learning outcomes

By the end of this chapter you should be able to:

- demonstrate understanding of the ways in which the Internet impacts on the provision of care;

- identify and critically review Internet sites of relevance to your field of practice;

- explain two ways in which the Internet can be used to improve patient care.

Introduction

The NHS Plan (DOH 2000) extended the rights of, and created new roles for, patients. The object was to enable patients to have a greater say in the provision of local health services and better access to information about their treatment (DOH 2003). One source of that information is the Internet. It is no longer unusual for patients to come to consultations with material they have downloaded and that they wish to discuss with professionals. Alternatively, patients can set up their own websites or use the Internet to discuss their health problems with others. The Internet provides an opportunity for patients to become better informed, which may in turn alter their relationships with professionals. However, not everything available on the Internet is accurate and patients need help in appraising the suitability and appropriateness of specific information for their circumstances.

The Internet is also a huge resource for professionals. For example, it provides educational opportunities for developing and sharing expertise in ways that are not constrained by distance or time zones. Virtual communities can be developed in which those with similar interests can share their ideas and learn from one another. The Internet poses challenges for professionals to adapt practice in ways that take account of the impact of the web on patient knowledge and expectations.

This chapter helps you to address both these issues through a set of exercises that will equip you to identify and evaluate some of the Internet-based information available to patients and provide you with skills that will inform the development of appropriate health education and promotion for those with both short-term and long-term health problems. The chapter then presents some ideas for ways in which the Internet can be used to inform and develop nursing practice.

Internet sites as a source of information

Searching for information about health-related subjects in academic libraries, databases and other sources has always been a slow and laborious task requiring patience, sophisticated skills and large amounts of time. Even those who possessed all three of these requirements would find that information was discovered in a rather piecemeal manner that was largely dependent on the range and quality of the sources available and an element of luck. Access to the Internet has revolutionised this situation, providing answers to questions within minutes rather than hours or years. Moreover, the breadth of information obtained will reflect a huge range of possibilities that draw on quite disparate and unrelated disciplines, which the manual searcher would find impossible to draw together. The routes to different items of information may also be very varied, thus taking the searcher along pathways that might otherwise remain unexplored. For example, patients seeking information about their medication may discover ideas that challenge those of their doctors or lead them to explore alternative therapies (Hardey 2001).

The Internet is available to everyone, although it may require some lateral thinking and creativity to locate whatever is required. What seems to matter is having the confidence to try and regular opportunities to practise. Searching for information is easily slotted into a busy work schedule and perceived as a normal part of the working day. In contrast, visiting a library requires a special journey, away from the workplace, to a setting that may not be experienced as welcoming or helpful (Tod *et al.* 2003; Hardey 2001).

The Internet can empower users to become more knowledgeable about their conditions, an outcome that is consistent with current health policy regarding the development of expert patients (DOH 2001a). This policy is aimed at those with long-term health problems, enabling them to take more control over and responsibility for the management of their condition. Patients are to be invited to undertake an expert patient course where they will have the opportunity to meet others with the same condition. Thus patients can learn from one another's experiences as well as through the facilitation of the course tutor. A pilot scheme was completed in August 2004. Findings from the evaluation of this scheme indicated that expert patients were better able to manage symptoms and felt more prepared for consultations with professionals. Alongside these experiences was a corresponding decrease in unnecessary GP and out-patient appointments as well as inappropriate attendances at A&E departments. Consequently, the scheme will be introduced into all Primary Care Trusts by 2008 via local delivery plans as part of an overall strategy for the management of long-term conditions (DOH 2005). This strategy is based on a model based on early detection of such conditions and the instigation of approaches to care designed to minimise complications. These approaches include the empowerment of patients and the promotion of self-care by proactive healthcare teams that can anticipate problems and work to avert crises.

> ## Over to you
>
> Visit www.expertpatients.nhs.uk.
> What is the aim of this scheme?
> What do you see as the possible benefits and disadvantages?

Clearly the Internet will play a part in enabling expert patients to continue to develop their expertise both as a source of information and as a way of monitoring their condition in ways that reduce the need for professional input. Some may even wish to become tutors for future courses so that gradually patients themselves, rather than professionals, facilitate the development of more expert patients. While this may be useful, in that people who directly experience a condition are often better placed to suggest strategies that help in the management of problems such as pain or depression, it is not intended that expert patients should replace professional expertise but rather that they should engage in a more collaborative relationship to ensure good disease management. This means that members of both parties must be aware of their limitations. Professionals must realise that they no longer have a monopoly over knowledge or understanding, while patients need to be aware that the Internet does not discriminate in providing access to information. Anything and everything is available but quality and accuracy cannot be guaranteed (Hardey 2001).

> ## Over to you
>
> Read Forkner-Dunn, J. (2003) 'Internet-based patient self-care: the next generation of health care delivery', *Journal of Medical Internet Research* 5 (2) article e6, available at www.jmir.org/2003/2/e8/.
> What does the author say about
> - using the Internet to monitor blood sugar levels in diabetes?
> - the impact of the Internet on the patient–professional relationship?

- The Internet is a resource for educating professionals and patients, and sharing experiences and information.

- Access to the Internet has changed the traditional relationships between patients and health care professionals because patients can gain access to a wide range of information.

- The expert patient scheme is intended to complement professional roles by helping those with long-term conditions to:

  - become better informed about their health problems;

  - manage their health problems more independently;

  - engage in self-help and self-care.

Evaluating Internet sites

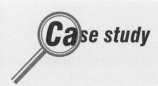

Case study

Joseph Ganley, aged 26, is a solicitor specialising in computer-based fraud. He was well until two weeks ago when he began to experience intermittent blurring of his vision, severe headaches and nausea that have necessitated treatment in the local A&E Department. Investigations have revealed the presence of an unusual form of brain tumour for which surgery is required. However, it is not clear whether Joseph will make a full recovery from this surgery. His parents are very concerned and have used the Internet to locate further information about this type of tumour and how it should be treated.

Joseph is meeting with the consultant and specialist nurse to discuss his treatment. He has brought with him details of two sites that both provide possible treatments. He wishes to discuss these and make a decision about the type of treatment that will be most appropriate for him.

Site A is based in Canada and offers a new drug that, it is claimed, will be as effective as the surgery. The drug costs $375 for three doses and a course of 25 doses is recommended. Other products are also advertised on the site and claim to enhance the effects of the drug. The drug and other products are supplied in powder form to be administered via intravenous infusion.

Site B is based in Brazil and presents a series of research reports about the introduction of a particular drug regimen for use alongside the type of surgery proposed for Joseph. The site is available in English and Portuguese. It offers links to the medical journals in which the papers have been published and email addresses are available for the main researchers.

How should the professionals react to this situation?

What advice should be given to Joseph?

Identify questions you might ask to help you evaluate a health-related website.

Joseph is justifiably concerned about what may happen to him as a result of surgery, particularly as his tumour is so rare. What matters most in this consultation is the response from professionals. An open-minded approach that enables individuals both to learn something new and to discard ideas that are no longer relevant will help to ensure dialogue rather than confrontation with Joseph. Treating his questions and ideas with respect, being open about professional concerns and exploring them with him rather than telling him what to do will facilitate progress towards concordance in which he and the professionals feel satisfied with the outcome.

As an expert in computer fraud he may well be aware of the potential of the Internet in all walks of life, but he may not be accustomed to looking critically at the content of sites relating to health issues. Concerns about both the quality and accuracy of such sites have prompted health professionals to redirect their evaluative skills. As yet there appears to be no definitive tool that covers every aspect of Internet site evaluation, but nevertheless there are some key factors to consider. The first concerns content. This should be both accurate and up to date. Some sites indicate when they were last updated, but there is no requirement for this to be done. Thus, in Joseph's case, the professionals may wish to query whether the information is recent, for example when the papers on site B were published, in order to determine whether the ideas put forward are consistent with current practice. While professionals will have more access than many patients to sources of advice and expertise that can help to verify the content of a site, it can sometimes be difficult to be confident about all the information provided, especially in highly specialised or rapidly developing fields. Consequently, it is good practice to draw on a range of sites and to compare information from different sources, from within the Internet and elsewhere, to assess accuracy (Kim *et al.* 1999; Liebermann 2000; Support 4 Learning available at www.support4learning.org.uk/reference/evaluate.htm). Thus the professionals in the case study might wish to spend some time with Joseph looking at sites A and B, perhaps comparing them with others and advising him about the potential advantages and disadvantages of relying on the Internet for health information. In particular, they might want to investigate the accuracy and truthfulness of site A.

The second group of factors to consider are concerned with responsibility for the site, including development and ownership. Both influence the presentation of the content. For example, sites belonging to public bodies, manufacturers or charities will inevitably present information in ways that reflect their overall aims. Such aims are usually fairly obvious even if they are not openly stated: to sell a product, to promote or implement a policy, to lobby for research or to promote self-help. Sites belonging to reputable sources, for example pharmaceutical companies or national organisations such as Diabetes UK (www.diabetes.org.uk), can usually be relied upon for truthfulness and accuracy, although they should never be used as the only source of information on any topic. However, other sites may give cause for concern. Site A may be genuine but could also be a scam to make money from those who feel frightened and desperate. Staff would have to explain to Joseph that even if he or his parents purchased the drug advertised, good professional practice would dictate that it could not be administered until it had been analysed to determine the contents. Sites owned and developed by individuals may be even less rigorous, reflecting very personal views that are not applicable to the majority. Such personal agendas may be far less easy to identify and may mislead people such as Joseph, and even some professionals, into thinking that the information presented is appropriate to their needs. It is therefore good practice to determine, where at all possible, not only who has produced the site but also who the intended users might be (Kim *et al* 1999; Liebermann 2000; Support 4 Learning available at www.support4learning.org.uk/reference/evaluate.htm).

A third set of factors concerns the ease with which the site can be accessed and used. Sites that are visually unattractive, slow to respond or complicated to use will not, even if they present accurate information, hold the visitor's interest. Alongside this issue it is useful to consider the security arrangements offered by those sites that collect personal data, with particular regard to clarifying who has access to that information and how it may be used (Kim *et al*. 1999; Liebermann 2000; Support 4 Learning available at www. support4learning.org.uk/reference/evaluate.htm). If, for example, Joseph's parents decided to buy some of the substances advertised by Site A, they might find that their credit card details and personal information are used for other purposes and could even find themselves the victims of fraud.

Finally, there are factors to consider about the international basis of the Internet. Specific treatments, products and devices may be available only in particular countries, each of which may vary in their mechanisms for controlling quality, especially in relation to new developments. Consequently, some treatments, products and devices may appear to have undergone more rigorous testing than is actually the case. For example, Site A may lead the reader to believe that the products have been thoroughly researched, but the site owners may be unable to provide any evidence of this. Alternatively,

Site A may be genuine. The items advertised may be very good but cost a lot of money to import. Patients like Joseph and their families could find themselves spending large sums on items that are not available through the NHS and, having once begun, then experience financial difficulties in meeting the costs involved and additional problems if they reach a point at which they are no longer able to afford them (Kim *et al* 1999; Liebermann 2000; Support 4 Learning available at www.support4learning.org.uk/reference/evaluate.htm). An additional factor to consider is that of language. The papers on Site B are available in English and Portuguese, but professionals would need to ascertain the language in which the papers were first written and then consider whether it is possible that changes may have been introduced by the process of translation. Translation is more than the substitution of one set of vocabulary by another. It requires the translator to have an understanding of the conventions that surround the way in which people communicate in the two languages involved and the expressions they might use to convey concepts. The translator has sometimes to encapsulate meaning rather than repeat it word for word and, consequently, slight variations may occur that could make a difference to practice (Hatton 1992).

Key points Top tips

- Professionals need to adapt their evaluative skills to review Internet sites in terms of:
    - suitability and appropriateness for patients and colleagues;
    - accuracy and currency of the content;
    - ownership of the site and the intended aims or function;
    - user-friendliness and security;
    - relevance to UK health care practice.
- Professionals need to be open-minded in their dealings with patients who wish to incorporate ideas from the Internet into their treatment and care.
- Professional willingness to listen and discuss new ideas forms a good basis for concordance.

Using the Internet to share good practice

Using the Internet tends to be a solitary activity. Individuals search for the information they require, use it for their own benefit but do not share it with others in any systematic way. Professionals need to move beyond this individualised activity to explore creatively ways in which the Internet can be integrated into everyday practice. If this can be achieved, then using the web will become part of the *socially embedded expertise* of the team (Benner *et al.* 1996). This term refers to the ways in which practitioners share ideas and information that are not to be found in formal sources such as textbooks or courses. This type of knowledge is important because patients' problems often do not conform to the ideas put forward in these sources. Practitioners need 'an active synthesis of skill, an art of practice which goes beyond established boundaries' (Schön 1983 p. 19) and that takes into account the individual situation of each patient. This means that, as well as theoretical knowledge, or **knowing how**, practitioners use practical knowledge or **knowing that** (Benner 1984).

Practical knowledge is shared informally. While the handover reports provide formal opportunities for communication, a great deal of exchange takes place while people are doing other activities. For example, McGee (2000) found that ward-based nurses shared information in narrative forms based on particular experiences such as 'what happened on the late shift last night' or 'the cardiac arrest incident yesterday'. These stories allowed nurses to review their experiences, learn from them and share their learning with others. Sharing and learning were, therefore, social rather than formal activities and became part of a ward team's collective knowledge and expertise. Thus incorporating information and learning from the Internet into the social exchanges within the team provides one approach to disseminating and using web-based information.

Over to you

Visit the intranet site in the organisation in which you currently work.

What types of information does the site provide?

Is there an in-house journal/newsletter? What format does it take?

Is there a forum through which good ideas about nursing practice can be shared across the Trust?

Over to you

Visit the Royal College of Nursing (RCN) website at www.rcn.org.uk.

Click on 'specialisms' and then 'children and young people'.

Make brief notes about the most recent news item.

How many forums address the needs of children and young people?

Select one forum and make brief notes about the latest news item.

Repeat this exercise by selecting a specialism related to your field of practice.

Keywords

Clinical governance

'A framework through which NHS organisations are accountable for continuously improving the quality of their services and safeguarding high standards of care by creating an environment in which excellence in clinical care will flourish' (DOH 1998 p. 3).

A more formal mechanism for sharing good practice arises from **clinical governance** and clinical practice benchmarking (DOH 1998, 2001b), which have led to an increased emphasis on evidence-based practice and standards of care (see pp. 154–61). The benchmarking cycle requires teams of practitioners to identify standards for specific aspects of practice and to compare and contrast their practice with that in another setting. Initially practitioners may choose to undertake this comparison locally, but some will be unable to do so because their work is highly specialised. Others may see advantages in looking outside the area to gain fresh perspectives on their work. The Internet offers the potential to develop and share ideas about standards and good practice between teams of nurses that would otherwise never meet. This potential is so far unexplored, but possible ways forward include compiling short reports that include video clips to demonstrate particular approaches to practice such as the prevention of pressure ulcers or the maintenance of safety. Alternatively a time-limited on-line discussion could be used to address problematic aspects of practice. These are suggestions only, and further work is needed to explore other ways in which the Internet might help in sharing practice.

Finally, the Internet offers opportunities for professionals to broaden their range of discourse and contacts as a means of sharing and learning from one another. One way of doing this is through discussion networks such as Minority Ethnic Health. This is a UK-wide network for those working with or researching among minority ethnic groups in health, social care, local government and other settings (contact minority-ethnic-health@ jiscmail.ac.uk). Membership is free and enables members to find out and keep abreast of developments in all aspects of practice and research.

Key points Top tips

- The Internet provides a vehicle for sharing good practice.
- Professional knowledge has theoretical and practical dimensions.
- Practical knowledge is shared informally.
- Internet-based knowledge could be incorporated into informal sharing systems.
- Work-based intranets, web-based professional forums and discussion networks provide ways through which good practice can be shared.
- Professional teams could explore the possibilities offered by the Internet for comparing and contrasting clinical practice benchmarking.

Using the Internet to help patients

A second approach to using the Internet is to exploit the potential of the web for patient education and support by helping patients to identify appropriate sites. Initially this may be done on an individual basis, but over time it should be possible for nursing teams to develop a database of sites that they can recommend to patients and their families. This database could be made available on the Internet, with hard copies provided alongside, or as part of, other patient literature.

Theory into Practice

Evaluating Internet sites

Select a specific health problem such as coronary heart disease, diabetes, arthritis, asthma, a communicable disease or some other illness that is relevant to your field of practice. Identify three different Internet sites that deal with this health problem. Try to ensure that these are aimed at different groups of people. For example, you might select one aimed at patients, another at nurses and a third that is intended for parents. Now complete the following table:

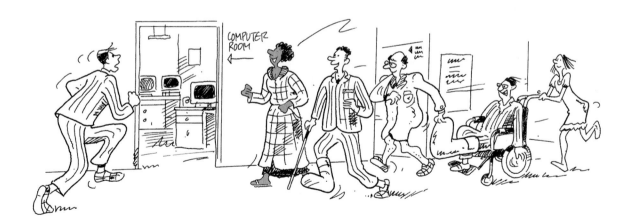

	Site 1	Site 2	Site 3
Content, e.g. What information does the site provide? Is the information accurate? How can it be checked? Is the information up to date? When was the site last updated?			
Ownership, e.g. Who/which organisation owns the site? What are their aims? What might be the implications of these aims for the content of the site?			
Audience, e.g. Is the site intended for patients, relatives, professionals?			
Security, e.g. Does the site ask for any personal information? What safeguards are in place to protect this information?			
User friendliness, e.g. How easy is it to use this site? What features are attractive and why? What features are unattractive and why?			
International aspects, e.g. What treatments, products and devices are promoted by the site? Are these available through the NHS? What is the price (in £) of the treatment, product or device concerned?			

Using the following key, score each site in relation to the topics set out below.
5 = excellent 4 = good 3 = average 2 = below average 1 = poor

	Site 1	Site 2	Site 3
Accurate content			
Up-to-date content			
Possible bias in content			
Security of personal information			
User friendliness			
Promotes treatments, products, devices available through the NHS			

Outline the advice you would give to patients and relatives/carers about each of the three sites that you have evaluated.

Alternatively, nursing teams may decide to develop their own website. This may be particularly helpful to patients requiring surgical treatment in a particular hospital or for those with conditions for which no self-help organisation exists.

Refle**Reflective activity**

Select one patient group for which you provide care.

What would be the advantages and disadvantages of designing a website for members of this group in the organisation in which you work?

Advantages

Developing a local website can be an inexpensive way of providing information about a specific aspect of health care practice because the organisation's server can provide ready-made access to the Internet. Thus teams will not be charged for setting up a site that is part of the organisation's business. Access to in-house IT expertise can help to create websites that are attractive, user friendly and informative. A website can provide a useful means of conveying to patients what to expect in relation to surgical procedures or other treatments. For example, local practice with regard to pre- and post-operative care can be explained and frequently asked questions can be easily addressed. Moreover, professionals will have control over the accuracy and currency of information provided. They will also be able to guide patients towards other appropriate sites and thus complement resources that are already available and incorporate relevant health education or health promotion messages.

Developing a website will also provide a means of actively involving service users in health care. Patients who are undergoing treatment or who have completed a treatment could be invited to participate. Their experiences will provide valuable insight into the types of information that other patients will find most useful, how that information can best be presented and the additional support they may require. Thus involving patients as service users has the potential to transform the quality of information available and, perhaps, challenge stereotypical thinking among professionals about what non-professionals may or may not understand.

Disadvantages

Large organisations such as NHS Trusts are likely to have in-house procedures for the development of websites and require conformity to a specific style. This may be constraining or may simply take a long time to achieve if organisational systems are slow and cumbersome. In-house IT expertise may be difficult to access unless members of staff in that field have designated responsibilities to work with practitioners who wish to develop local websites. This may lead to frustration in designing and maintaining the site. In addition, practitioners will need to agree some responsibilities among themselves, particularly with regard to who will liaise with IT staff and who will ensure that the information given on the site is up to date. Practice changes over time and the site will, therefore, require regular checks to ensure that it is current. In any health care team there will be members of staff who seek to move in order to gain more experience. Thus team members may agree on how responsibilities are to be shared, only to find that individuals have left and that nothing has been done.

Conclusion

This chapter has helped you to think about the potential usefulness of the Internet in enhancing both professional practice and the information available to patients. The Internet offers many opportunities for sharing good practice through local intranet networks and national professional forums. It also offers the potential for practice-based teams to compare and contrast their work as part of the clinical practice benchmarking cycle. Patients too may benefit from the Internet, providing members of staff are open to new ideas and willing to discuss new or unfamiliar ideas about care. However, the vast amount of information available through the Internet varies considerably in quality and accuracy. Professionals, therefore, need to adapt the skills that enable them to evaluate critically other sources to reviewing websites applicable to their fields of practice. Patients and less experienced professionals require guidance about the use of the Internet with regard to health issues and the ways in which individuals can be misled.

ʀʀʀʀʀ**Rapid recap**

1 What is the aim of the expert patient scheme?
2 Briefly explain two ways in which the Internet may be used to share good practice.
3 What are the key points to remember in evaluating websites for health care?
4 Which two types of nursing knowledge have been outlined in this chapter? Briefly explain them.
5 What are the advantages of involving patients in designing a website?

References

Benner, P. (1984) *From Novice to Expert. Excellence and Power in Clinical Nursing Practice*. Menlo Park CA, Addison-Wesley.

Benner, P., Tanner, C. and Chesla, C. (1996) *Expertise in Nursing Practice. Caring, Clinical Judgement and Ethics*. New York, Springer Publishing Company.

Department of Health (DOH) (1998) *Clinical Governance. Quality in the NHS*. London, DOH.

Department of Health (DOH) (2000) *The NHS Plan. A Plan for Investment. A Plan for Reform*. London, DOH.

Department of Health (DOH) (2001a) *The Expert Patient: A New Approach to Chronic Disease Management for the 21st Century*. London, DOH.

Department of Health (DOH) 2001b) *The Essence of Care. Patient-focused Benchmarking for Health Care Practitioners*. London, DOH.

Department of Health (DOH) (2005) *Supporting People with Long Term Conditions. An NHS and Social Care Model to Support Local Innovation and Integration*. London, DOH.

Department of Health (DOH) (2003) Choice, Responsiveness and Equity in the NHS and Social Care. A National Consultation. London, DOH

Forkner-Dunn, J. (2003) 'Internet-based patient self-care: the next generation of health care delivery', *Journal of Medical Internet Research* 5 (2) article e6, available at www.jmir.org/2003/2/e8/.

Hardey, M. (2001) 'Doctor in the house: the Internet as a source of lay knowledge and the challenge to expertise', Chapter 68 in B. Davey, A. Gray and C. Seale (eds) *Health and Disease: A Reader*, 3rd edn. Buckingham, Open University Press, pp. 400–5.

Hatton, D. (1992) 'Information transmission in bilingual, bicultural contexts', *Journal of Community Health Nursing* 9 (1) pp. 53–9.

Kim, P., Eng, T. R., Deering, M. J. and Maxfield, A. (1999) 'Published criteria for evaluating health related websites: review', *British Medical Journal* 318 (6 March) pp. 647–9.

Liebermann, J. (2000) 'Evaluating health web sites', in *Consumer Health. An On Line Manual*. Available at http://nnlm.gov/scr/conhlth/evalsite.htm

McGee, P. (2000) *Culturally-sensitive Nursing: A Critique*. Unpublished PhD Thesis. Birmingham, University of Central England.

Schön, D. (1983) *The Reflective Practitioner. How Professionals Think in Action*. London, Avebury.

Tod, A. M., Harrison, J., Morris Docker, S., Black, R. and Wolstenholme, D. (2003) 'Access to the Internet in an acute care area: experiences of nurses', *British Journal of Nursing* 12 (7) pp. 425–34.

8

Care in the multidisciplinary team

Lynne Wigens

Learning outcomes

By the end of this chapter you should be able to:

- understand the concept of multidisciplinary teams and their potential;

- examine the advantages and disadvantages of collaborative styles of professional practice;

- explore the contribution of user perspectives to multidisciplinary working.

○━ᴇ *Keywords*

Multidisciplinary

A co-operative enterprise where the traditional forms and divisions of professional knowledge and authority are retained.

Interprofessional

Willingness to share and give up exclusive claims to specialised knowledge and authority if the needs of the patient can be met more efficiently by other professional groups (Owens *et al.* 1995).

Introduction

When someone requires health carer interventions they often face a whole range of health care workers who have different views and expertise. If each health care professional works independently the patient/service user may view their care as disjointed and less effective than it could have been, but if health care professionals work together within teams, these workers are more likely to meet patient needs. **Multidisciplinary** teams have, therefore, been identified as one of the ways in which health care delivery can be tailored to meet the needs of sick, disabled and vulnerable people. In fact, some research has gone as far as to indicate a link between staff working effectively within teams and reduced patient mortality (West *et al.* 2002).

With the emphasis on valuing patients and the increasing demand for patient care, 'providing a health care service requires several professionals to work together closely and continuously together, not just at an **interprofessional** liaison committee, but day-by-day in clinics, surgeries and hospitals' (Walby *et al.* 1994 p. 17).

Leathard (2003) refers to the 'terminological quagmire' that surrounds health care team working where 'multi', 'inter', 'disciplinary' and 'professional' are often used in various combinations. Sometimes the terms multidisciplinary and interprofessional are used interchangeably when talking about team working, but it can be useful to appreciate the differences between these two terms.

This chapter looks at care in the multidisciplinary team, but I would like to argue that multidisciplinary care is a stepping stone towards interprofessional team work, and much of the chapter content also applies to this.

Interprofessional collaboration has been identified as crucial to modernisation of the health service (DOH 2000a, 2000b). Within this chapter you will learn about changing professional roles, the reasons for and barriers to collaboration and the importance of service user involvement for true multidisciplinary team work. Activities and case studies will be used to explore the links between multidisciplinary team work, caring, productivity and creativity. Multidisciplinary working is now recognised as an essential curriculum component within education for health care professions, helping students to make the links between team work and professional practice. The team working skills learnt during the foundations of your professional training will stay with you, becoming part of who you are as a practitioner. So learning the importance of multidisciplinary working is one of the most significant ways to influence your caring practice.

The multidisciplinary team

Patients attending their GP surgery with a chest infection may interact with only a limited number of staff during the course of their illness, for example the receptionist, the GP and the pharmacist. These staff could be labelled as a patient-centred or 'intrinsic' multidisciplinary team. However, if we compare the number of health care practitioners involved in the next case, it becomes clear that co-ordination of interprofessional involvement is necessary for the most effective care to be delivered.

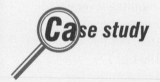

Case study

Jane Hawthorne, aged 67 and living alone since she was widowed two years ago, is soon to be discharged from hospital. She was admitted following an exacerbation of her chronic obstructive pulmonary disease when she became very breathless. She still requires some assistance with her daily activities, particularly mobilising and washing, and is taking a revised set of medications. Her care will require a 'full and functional team' approach where health care practitioners who deliver care need to review and share their information regarding her progress.

List the health practitioners who might be involved in Jane's care over the next two weeks, and the main components of their role. Do you see any situations where there could be duplication or overlaps in the care/treatment provided by different team members?

When you thought about the health care professionals who might be involved in Jane's care you probably identified staff within the hospital and also in the community. Outlined in Table 8.1 is the broad range of roles and responsibilities of some of the health carers you may have identified (although the list is clearly not exhaustive).

Table 8.1 Roles and responsibilities of health carers

Health care practitioner	Roles and responsibilities
Doctor (medical consultant and general practitioner)	The doctor is responsible for medical diagnosis, likely prognosis and pharmacological care. The medical remit is met through symptom identification, determining therapies, monitoring progress and agreeing future plans.
Nurse (ward based and community district nurses, including the practice nurse and respiratory nurse	The nurse assesses the patient's problems, plans, and implements, and evaluates care in relation to patient comfort, psychological support prevention of tissue damage, maintenance of specialist) nutrition, administration of drugs, and monitoring elimination and vital functions. The nurse is frequently the co-ordinator of care, liaising with a range of other health care professionals.
Physiotherapist (hospital and community based)	The physiotherapist is mainly concerned with the clinical assessment of physical disorders that affect a patient's mobility or physical functioning. As well as delivering treatments/exercises the physiotherapist encourages the patient to become mobile and gain maximum functioning.
Occupational therapist (OT) (hospital and community based)	The occupational therapist undertakes a detailed assessment of cognitive and physical functioning in relation to all the activities of daily living, e.g. dressing, eating and using the bath or shower. The OT investigates the patient's domestic circumstances, e.g. suitability of accommodation and family support available.
Pharmacist	The pharmacist manages all aspects of the use of medicine, working so that these medicines are used safely and effectively. The pharmacist interacts with patients and other health care practitioners so that the right medicine in the appropriate presentation is dispensed to the right patient at the right time.
Social worker	The social worker is involved in assessing the patient's home situation and needs. If there are any social problems that can affect health care, this will be dealt with by the social worker, e.g. arranging residential care, financial issues if there are no relatives to assist, benefits advice and housing. The social worker also determines access to social care facilities such as meals-on-wheels and day centre attendance.

Although the table refers to qualified/registered health care professionals, it is important to appreciate the role of support, carer or assistant grades within the multidisciplinary team. **Skill mix** involves professionals being willing to accept a form of interprofessional working that recognises the possibility that some needs may be met more effectively by lesser-trained staff.

Changes in skill mix are usually brought about through delegation, substitution or diversification (Adams *et al.* 2000). The three main forms of skill mix are:

- mix of skills across different health disciplines involved in delivering a service;
- mix of skills held within a particular discipline (including trained staff and associated support staff);
- mix of skills held by an individual.

In the following excerpt from a discussion with a practice nurse, she talks about how skill mix helped her surgery meet the challenges of the Coronary Heart Disease National Service Framework:

> We wanted to free up more of the practice nurse's time to concentrate on primary prevention of CHD [coronary heart disease] and heart failure through linking in with the GP reviews of these patients. It was made possible through us employing a health care assistant who learnt to do phlebotomy, blood pressure checks and ECG [electrocardiogram] recordings. Although there were some concerns at first this new role has really made a difference to patient care.

As well as support roles being important in care, some patients will also require specialist staff who have narrower but equally important roles and responsibilities in relation to the care of certain patients. In the previous case study, for example, Jane may well have received care from a specialist respiratory nurse.

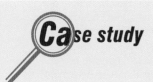

Case study

Mr Davies is receiving treatment and care for bowel cancer. He has become confused about the roles of the range of nurses who are involved in his care.

How might you explain the different roles of the nurse endoscopist, district nurse, stoma nurse, oncology nurse specialist and the Macmillan nurse to Mr Davies?

Through answering the question related to this case study, it becomes clear that even within one profession there are many specialist roles. Your answer probably looked something like this:

- A nurse endoscopist is a registered nurse who has undergone additional training to perform a diagnostic procedure (in the case study above, sigmoidoscopy).
- A district nurse is a generalist who provides individual packages of care within the community.
- The stoma nurse meets the patient prior to undergoing an operation (in the case study above, a colostomy) to site the best position for the stoma, and helps care for the stoma in the initial post-operative period progressing patient education towards self-care.
- An oncology nurse specialist explains the chemotherapy treatments and administers these.
- The Macmillan nurse who is based in the community offers specialist psychological support, practical advice, skills in pain management and advice on treatment options.

So within a multidisciplinary team there are generalists, support roles and often specialist roles as necessary. The broad remits of three examples of multidisciplinary teams are identified below together with details of (1) the key health professional, (2) the support staff and (3) examples of specialist staff who may comprise the membership of these multidisciplinary teams:

Primary health care teams These teams are responsible for promoting and maintaining the health of people in their local community. These needs are met by:

1 general practitioners, community nurses, practice nurses, social workers and clinical support staff;
2 practice managers, administrative staff, voluntary staff;
3 public health practitioners, child protection specialists.

Community mental health teams These teams are responsible for community-based services for people with mental health problems or illnesses. These needs are met by:

1 psychiatrists, community psychiatric nurses, clinical psychologists, social workers and their associated clinical support staff;
2 administrative staff, voluntary staff;
3 assertive outreach psychiatric services staff, substance abuse specialist nurses.

Breast cancer teams These teams are responsible for the diagnosis and treatment of breast cancer, crossing hospital and community based care. The needs of breast care patients are met by:

1 medical consultants (range of specialities including breast surgeons and medical oncologists), breast care nurses, radiographers (therapy);

2 administrative staff, voluntary staff, patient support groups;

3 genetic counsellors, plastic surgeons.

When you identify the number of roles and people potentially involved in the care of one patient with breast cancer (which includes the breast cancer team and ward and community general staff) it becomes clear that effort needs to be invested in developing a team approach that is effective.

Key points Top tips

- Multidisciplinary working has become increasingly important as patient care has become more complex and modernised.
- Skill mix is frequently undertaken in determining staffing decisions, and assistant practitioners working in support roles to health care professionals are often part of the interprofessional team.
- There are increasing numbers of specialist roles developing within health care.

Multidisciplinary team development

A team is a group of people who share common objectives and who need to work together to achieve these. Three types of need are present in every team:

- individual
- group
- task.

The length of time spent on each of these needs within the team depends on many variables, a major one being the stage of the team's development.

Over time, the provision of the health service has generated hundreds of different specialities and professions, resulting in the requirement for subtle and complex decision-making processes. Health care professionals are often working in uncertain and complex situations, and individual cases require assessment and support from a range of staff with well-developed knowledge and skills. Effective teams do not develop overnight, and teams will often go through stages in their development.

Team development stages

There are often four stages in the development of a team:

Stage 1   Orientation, testing and dependency stage. During this stage, individual needs are dominant as individuals try to find out whether their personal needs will be met.

Stage 2   Intra-conflict stage. During this stage the emphasis is on meeting team and individual needs. Team needs include such things as ground rules, team structure and modes of communicating. Little work gets done in either this or the previous stage.

Stage 3   Team cohesion. In this stage a bit more time is spent on the task, but the bulk of the time is spent on team needs, while less time is spent on individual needs.

Stage 4   Problem solving and interdependence. During this stage approximately equal amounts of time are spent on individual, team and task needs.

Although it is useful to understand the stages in team development, it is important to realise that you can be a member of many teams, and that teams can be transient in nature. For example, the physiotherapist joining a ward team during a ward round becomes part of this team for a short period of time and then goes back to their physiotherapy/rehabilitation team.

Over to you

Identify a team that you are currently a member of (it does not need to be a health care team), and describe the purpose of this team's existence.

List the personal needs you have as they relate to being a member of this team.

List your perception of the needs you all share as members of this team.

Identify the tasks of this team.

Identify the developmental stage your team is at.

When you thought about your team in the last activity you might have thought back to when the team first got together. Team members need to spend time getting to know each other if their team work is to be effective, but there may be little apparent time to do this within a busy clinical environment. Although it might be good for members of a multidisciplinary team to spend time getting to know each other in a sociable way, more realistically this might be achieved through a common group activity, such as setting time

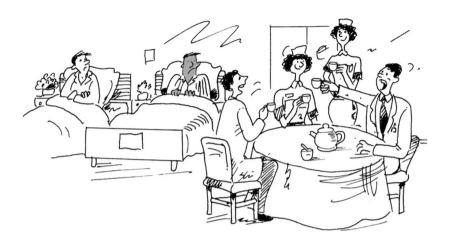

aside to develop a protocol or undertake a case review. This shared learning activity can help to promote team cohesion.

The effectiveness of team work, Bruce (1980) suggests, can be identified as nominal, convenient or committed. These terms are defined as follows:

- nominal team – where there is only very limited teamwork occurring;

- convenient team – where a clinician (often the doctor) delegates work to other health care practitioners;

- committed team – where the team members invest time and energy into their team work.

Over to you

Here are some questions you might ask a few members of a multidisciplinary team. Which term (nominal, convenient or committed) might best describe the type of team within which they currently work?

- Are you happy working in your team?
- Do you think other team members are happy?
- Is the team committed to the work?
- Is the team good at adapting to change?
- Do you all continue to learn together?
- Is the team allowing you to personally develop?

What other things could you do, apart from asking questions, to ascertain the level of team work?

- Teams develop over time through their interactions.
- Team development can progress through different stages, from orientation to intra-conflict, on to team cohesion and finally problem solving and interdependence.
- The effectiveness of teams can be variable, ranging from nominal or limited team working to committed team working.

What encourages multidisciplinary teamwork?

There are a number of factors that have been found to help in the development of multidisciplinary teams. These include:

- personal commitment
- sharing a common goal
- clarity of roles
- good lines of communication
- institutional support
- leadership.

Personal commitment

If some of the members of a multidisciplinary team have past favourable experiences of this way of working, they can argue for this method of working in the new setting. Interprofessional team work needs committed champions who share their vision and make working together a reality, using their networks and clinical practice experience (Pirrie *et al.* 1998). The value placed on making regular contact with patients can affect nurses' perceptions of other individual health care professionals, meaning that stronger alliances are made with staff who spend time on a regular basis with patients, as hands-on clinicians are viewed as more likely to put work into multidisciplinary working. Interprofessional working has seen the emergence of new coalitions between health care professions and new ways of working in practice settings. Nurses and other health care professionals have been found to work on the development of sound relationships with other professionals (Pirrie *et al.* 1998).

Sharing a common goal

Successful multidisciplinary teams are likely to have invested time in developing a shared vision about the service and to have a clear idea as to the objectives they are all working towards. Having a shared vision is, therefore, linked to teams having committed team members. This is in evidence where teams set themselves stretching quality targets and challenges around innovative practice (West *et al*. 2002). The common goal and shared objectives need to integrate with those of the patient/service user as part of the multidisciplinary team. Teams should comprise those who have the skills to meet the patient's/service user's specific needs, and increasingly specialised professions need to be able to respond to and treat the patient as a whole human being. One challenge is to create effective helping strategies that recognise the patient as a thinking and feeling person who is an integral part of a complex network of multidisciplinary relationships.

The patient/service user needs to be at the centre and integral to the multidisciplinary team. Empowerment has been defined as the process of helping people to assert control over the factors that affect their lives, and it requires power sharing in the health care context. Patient empowerment is a goal strongly linked to perceived inequalities in the relationships of patients to health carers, and multidisciplinary teams need to place increased emphasis on health promotion, allowing individuals to take greater responsibility for their own health. Patients who have a greater control over decisions and the ability to change their behaviours can significantly affect their health outcomes. This involves team members securing and using resources that promote and foster a sense of control, and accepting the situation when patients choose to reject professional help.

Clarity of roles

The boundaries between professional groups tend to be maintained through claims of competence in dealing with different problems, and it is these differences and similarities that are often stressed during initial training. Identification with a professional group leads to an ability to determine insiders and outsiders and what counts as the central work domain. Multidisciplinary team work does not require all members of staff to undertake the same roles, but it is essential that roles are clear. As health care professionals develop, they may expand their areas of practice, and team members need opportunities to gain insight into the changing boundaries of each other's practice.

In the quote below a midwife talks about how her professional boundary changed:

I was a hospital-based midwife, but over the past year we have been reorganised into a 'group-practice' midwifery team. Seven of us have been joined in a team that looks after around two hundred and fifty women covering a community locality. We

Keywords

Role-blurring
The capacity to relinquish rigid concepts of one's professional role and a willingness to learn from other professionals.

take responsibility for these women from conception to the tenth post-natal day. This model of working has really challenged the boundaries of my practice, and I feel that I am now doing aspects of work that in the past would have been medical work.

Multidisciplinary team members need to have a degree of role confidence and to feel secure with their professional identity if they are to be comfortable with **role-blurring**.

Professional identity has been viewed as being integrated with the health carer's personal sense of identity and involves, for example, a feeling of being a nurse who can practise with skill, taking responsibility for one's own actions, while maintaining an awareness of one's attributes and limitations (Ohlen and Segesten 1998). The identity of a nurse – aligned to caring as a central component of the role – has had consequences for the image of nurses and nursing and interprofessional working. Difficulties can remain with regard to relationships with other professions, especially medicine, as medical professional bodies may reflect professional self-interest in limiting the expansion of advanced nursing and allied health professional roles.

For effective multidisciplinary working, nurses are learning to appreciate the caring roles of others. Professional identity develops though the interactions of individual nurses during their practice and changes over time as the practitioner becomes more experienced and works with other professionals.

Good lines of communication

Multidisciplinary functioning depends on decisions being taken by the team as a whole, not exclusively by one or two powerful members. It requires open communication between all involved professionals rather than the transmission of information in one direction only. Successful team work depends on the personalities, commitment and degree of flexibility of the team members, and calls for members to examine relationships in an honest and straightforward manner. Formal communication forums are required for staff to discuss working and patients with multidisciplinary team members present. Depending on the clinical area, case meetings, care conferences, ward rounds and multidisciplinary meetings are the settings in which decisions are made. Some agreed and formal understanding of key concepts is essential, for instance on confidentiality, an issue on which each health care professional may have their own unique understanding. It is a practical necessity for effective functioning that all team members should have an opportunity to contribute, and this should ideally be in a constructive environment where all contributions are valued.

Multidisciplinary documentation, accessed by all team members, can also assist in supporting interprofessional working. Developing and using the same documentation, e.g. an integrated care pathway (ICP), requires close communication between professionals and work towards a previously agreed common goal. An ICP is written by the multidisciplinary team and outlines the anticipated flow of care (assessment, planning, implementation and evaluation) for patients with a specific diagnosis, strengthening the team approach to decision-making. This method of managing patient care helps NHS organisations in their efforts to try to involve patients in decision-making about their care and to ensure that patients receive appropriate, high-quality and cost-effective care. Once an integrated care pathway is printed and in use, team members need only to record variation from the care pathway. Using an ICP makes it possible to identify reasons for delayed discharge and variances from normal, and improves written communication.

In applying their unique talents, multidisciplinary team members are able to express their views and ideas and take up opportunities for interprofessional supervision, coaching and feedback. Some disagreement is both inevitable and to be expected as the team members make efforts to understand the others' points of view. In addition to the formal communication structures, there is a need for strong informal communication between members; this can take the form of a chat, talking together and supportive conversations.

Institutional support

Improved interprofessional collaboration can lead to efficient use of staff resources, increased work satisfaction, and more integrated services (Forte 1997). Bearing this in mind, you might expect strong institutional support for multidisciplinary teams, but this can be variable. Team leaders and members need to learn ways of communicating effectively with managers and establishing common territory. A particular problem can be caused when team members are employees of different institutions, e.g. social care, hospital, community and mental health trusts. Joint planning and funding streams, and closer actual and virtual proximity of services, can aid interprofessional collaboration.

A movement to **boundaryless** or seamless care is considered part of the solution to effective multidisciplinary working, within the extent of professional expertise (Ashkenas *et al.* 1995). These boundaries can be:

⚷ *Keywords*

Boundaryless

The barriers or boundaries of practice e.g. between departments, are more permeable and open to cross boundary integrated working.

1 horizontal – between disciplines or departments within an institution;
2 vertical – between different levels with a hierarchy;
3 external – between different trusts, agencies and professional bodies;
4 psychological – individuals' feelings and emotions that affect teamwork.

Institutional support for new ways of working and a shared purpose are required for effective interprofessional working, not just the blurring of professional boundaries. Institutional support could be indicated by giving time for communication forums, and formalising the team or **community of practice** (Wenger *et al.* 2002) within the organisation.

The exploration by Wenger *et al.* (2002) of the relationships of communities of practice to their institutions identified five main relationships:
1 unrecognised or invisible;
2 bootlegged, and only visible informally to the circle of people in the know;
3 legitimised and officially sanctioned as valuable;
4 strategic and widely recognised as central to organisational success;
5 transformative, capable of redefining its environment.

As multidisciplinary teams develop, they may progress through these levels of relationships within their institutions. Team integration is the extent to which team members work together using their diverse knowledge and skills, but also how the team capitalises on their role within the wider institutional structures.

Leadership

A key issue for the multidisciplinary team is that of leadership, but this does not mean that leadership necessarily lies with only one member of the team. One or more individuals can provide leadership, but there needs to be clarity and no conflict about the leadership of the team if working is to be effective. Leaders within the multidisciplinary team are responsible for developing clear objectives, encouraging participation, focusing on quality and supporting innovation (West 2002). In contrast, managers are responsible for ensuring that people work together and that standards and targets are met.

A significant cultural shift is required for interprofessional working, and the time that clinical leaders spend with less experienced health care professionals at the start of their careers

⊶ᵣ *Keywords*

Community of practice
A group/team that develops their own team practices, routines, rituals, stories and histories. Newcomers learn membership through social interactions with existing team members.

can be a unique opportunity to impact on future interprofessional working. Effective interprofessional leadership helps develop communication channels and a team spirit across the professions. Encouraging the gradual development of interpersonal support that extends beyond the workplace can also contribute to a team feeling. Learning about other health care professionals within the multidisciplinary team involves not just an understanding of their role but knowing and valuing them as authentic people (Wigens 2004). When this has been achieved, it can reduce the stress around interprofessional working and increase respect for each other's unique contribution to patient care (Nolan 1995). As a result, more time will be allocated to engage in multiprofessional working. The strength of interprofessional relationships and working is related to leadership vigour and networking.

Key points | Top tips

- There are many factors that help in the development of teams, including personal commitment to effective multidisciplinary team working.
- Multidisciplinary teams require management support and a willingness to blur professional boundaries.
- Communication and clinical leadership are crucial for effective interprofessional working.

What factors can inhibit multidisciplinary teamwork?

The sometimes contested nature of interprofessional working often revolves around the nature of the professions (their skills, knowledge and values) and the object of their interventions (areas of the patient's life in which they intervene). Despite the strong support at a national level for multidisciplinary team work within health care, evidence continues to indicate that this is being adopted with varying levels of success. Some factors that can inhibit interprofessional teamwork include:

- attitudes of team members;
- time and resource constraints;
- the differing professional bodies.

Attitudes of team members

If one or more of the team members is unconvinced about the advantages of multidisciplinary working, or even opposed to it, this can severely affect the co-ordination of care delivery. Opposition to team work can be based on misinformation, stereotypes held of other health care professions and past experiences. This can be particularly problematic if the members who are opposed to team working are in a position of authority. With true interprofessional working, authority is devolved downwards to the team level, and this can, potentially, reduce the influence of professions (e.g. medical professions) that operate through hierarchical structures.

A potent source of conflict in multidisciplinary teams can be the wide variety of professional backgrounds of members, and through **professional socialisation** individuals may bring with them their preconceptions, assumptions, stereotyped attitudes and traditional rivalries.

Professional hierarchies and feelings of domination by other professions can cause tribalism (Becher 1994). The knowledge of another health care professional is gathered through a series of encounters and can be biased or selectively remembered (Eraut 2000). Appreciation of the importance of context to relationships, and the possible risks of bias, have great relevance to interprofessional working.

○━ฅ *Keywords*

Professional socialisation

The process that a student health care practitioner undergoes during their education to acquire the skills, attitudes, values and outlooks that are deemed to constitute a particular professional role.

> ## *Over to you*
>
> Choose one of the following health care professions (pick one that you encounter less often during your work):
>
> - dietician
> - social worker
> - podiatrist
> - speech and language therapist
> - radiographer.
>
> Write the name of the profession in the centre of a blank sheet of A4 paper. Now write any words that come into your head when you think of this profession (uncensored), connecting each by a line to the word in the centre. When you have finished, analyse what you have written, and think about what informed your biases and assumptions.

Different health professions have varying levels of autonomy and specialisation, and this can inhibit communication. A power imbalance within a multidisciplinary team can act as a barrier to collaboration, and the legal power of doctors regarding medical diagnosis can be used as a justification to rule over clinical decisions (Lockhart-Wood 2000). The nurse–doctor relationship has been viewed as essentially patriarchal, with the notion that nursing as caring is an extension of the female role, although it has been acknowledged that what might appear to be unproblematic subordination is more likely to involve a considerable nursing input into decision-making (Porter 1992). Although a team may talk of wonderful, idealistic notions of collective working through mutually agreed goals, shared and flexible leadership, and a genuine blurring and overlapping of roles, in reality this is often not the case.

Time and resource constraints

There are logistical reasons why multidisciplinary teamwork can be inhibited. If there are staff shortages, it can prove difficult to support interprofessional activities that are time consuming. Organising and attending meetings when all members can be available can be problematic, particularly when such events take staff away from their care delivery work. Accommodation for meetings may be limited, and geographical distances between staff can add to the pressures of everyday working. Access to evidence to underpin practice decisions may also be limited by the availability of information technology and library resources.

Although multidisciplinary team work helps in ensuring more effective use of the individual and team resources (including experience and skills), and allows easier access to an accurate assessment of the patient's needs, it does require time for team development. Overall, multidisciplinary working helps resolve the problems inherent in increasing specialisation when there is also a strong call for holistic models of care, but it does require institutional support that can be lacking when an institution is financially stretched.

In some instances where interprofessional collaboration has been viewed as essential, and there is a risk that resource constraints may hinder this, mandated governmental standards have been put in place to influence this. An example of this has been in the area of child protection, where care is often delivered across a range of agencies that need to work closely together.

The differing professional bodies

Health care professionals must work within their accountability and legal framework. The Nursing and Midwifery Council and the Health Professions Council have a responsibility for protecting patients and maintaining a register of health professionals, setting standards of education and training and proficiency, and investigating complaints. When professionals work collaboratively they must constantly review whether they are acting within the rule of law and whether, if they perform a task previously done by another health care professional, this is done to the same standard (the rule of negligence). Considerable work has been undertaken to give guidance to professionals about moving their boundaries of work (e.g. NMC *Code of Professional Conduct* 2002), but this can still create obstacles to collaborative working.

The boundaries between the work of doctors and that of nurses and allied health professions are changing, with these staff taking over aspects of junior doctors' clinical work. New territory for nurses appears to have taken different directions according to the clinical areas in which they work. In general wards nurses are carving out an expanded area of influence and decision-making by assuming responsibility for the social care of patients and communication with relevant outside agencies. However, in the specialised clinical areas nurses are claiming a stake in the cure terrain by taking on new technical-medical tasks.

Case study

The community dietician has developed a dietician-led coeliac clinic. On a regular (around six-monthly) basis the dietician meets individuals who have been diagnosed as having coeliac disease. At the clinic the dietician checks compliance with the diet through patient questioning and a detailed dietary history-taking.

What obstacles/hindering factors can you identify that might reduce the effectiveness of this health care practitioner-led clinic (or any other)?

Key points | Top tips

- Barriers to interprofessional working include the attitudes of team members, time and resource constraints and the differing professional bodies.
- An appreciation of factors that hinder interprofessional working can help in attempts to make service improvements.

Interprofessional education

Effective interprofessional working has been linked to the development of interprofessional educational curricula, which are seen as crucial to stop the seeds of division being sown in profession-specific education programmes. These divisions may then be perpetuated in practice and reinforced by professional bodies and differing working conditions. In a study of clinical nurse specialists' interaction with other health care professionals, Arslanian-Engoren (1995) concluded that the educational preparation of the nurse was a key aspect in supporting collaboration.

Interprofessional education is an umbrella term for multidisciplinary learning, interdisciplinary learning, shared learning, common learning and multiprofessional education. Interprofessional education incorporates the arrangements made for people from different disciplines/professions to learn with each other, and it has been suggested that the term interprofessional encompasses professions learning from and about each other to improve collaboration, rather than just learning side by side (Centre for the Advancement of Interprofessional Education (CAIPE) 1997). Interprofessional learning promotes teamwork and cultivates collaborative practice.

There are logistical difficulties in organising and delivering interprofessional educational programmes (Pirrie *et al.* 1998). Placing professionals together in multidisciplinary learning groups does not necessarily guarantee the development of a shared understanding. For instance, student nurses who shared lectures with medical and allied health professional students in their first year did not appear to develop an enthusiastic approach to multidisciplinary working. Student nurses often sat in segregated groups and expressed concerns about the lack of opportunities to consolidate their own sense of professional identity before the introduction of interprofessional education within their programme (Pirrie *et al.* 1998).

Interprofessional education is happening in a wide range of health care programmes at pre- and post-qualification levels.

Reflective activity

Reflect on the interprofessional elements of your health care course, and determine how these have affected your views about multidisciplinary team working.

Conclusion

Throughout this chapter I have argued that interprofessional learning impacts on patient care in a positive way. This is supported by evidence of improved knowledge and raised skill levels (Hammick 2000). Interprofessional education and training is likely to be beneficial to future multidisciplinary working, and when combined with an awareness of the factors that facilitate multidisciplinary team development, the future for interprofessional team working looks good.

> ## RRRRR*Rapid recap*
>
> 1 What are the three main forms of skill mix?
> 2 Define the word 'team' and list the types of need that are present in every team.
> 3 List the four stages of team development.
> 4 List four factors that have been found to help in the development of multidisciplinary teams.
> 5 Identify and briefly outline three factors that can inhibit interprofessional team work.

References

Adams, A., Lugsden, E., Chase, J., Arber, S. and Bond, S. (2000) 'Skill-mix change and work intensification in nursing', *Work, Employment and Society* 14 pp. 541–5.

Arslanian-Engoren, C. (1995) 'Lived experiences of clinical nurse specialists who collaborate with physicians: a phenomenological study', *Clinical Nurse Specialist* 9 (2) pp. 68–74.

Ashkenas, R., Ulrich, D., Prahalad, C. and Jick, T. (1995) *The Boundaryless Organization: Breaking the Chains of Organizational Structure*. San Francisco CA, Jossey-Bass.

Becher, T. (1994) 'The significance of disciplinary differences', *Studies in Higher Education* 19 (2) pp. 151–61.

Bruce, N. (1980) *Teamwork for Preventative Care*. Research Studies Press. Chichester, John Wiley and Sons.

Centre for the Advancement of Interprofessional Education (CAIPE) (1997) *Interprofessional Education – a Definition*. London, CAIPE.

Department of Health (DOH) (2000a) *The NHS Plan: a Plan for Investment, a Plan for Reform*. London, DOH, HMSO.

Department of Health (DOH) (2000b) *A Health Service for All the Talents: Developing the NHS Workforce – Consultation Paper*. London, DOH, HMSO.

Eraut, M. (2000) 'Non-formal learning and tacit knowledge in professional work', *British Journal of Educational Psychology* 70 pp. 113–36.

Forte, P. (1997) 'The high cost of conflict', *Nursing Economics* 15 (3) pp. 119–23.

Hammick, M. (2000) 'Interprofessional education: evidence from the past to guide the future', *Medical Teacher* 22 pp. 472–8.

Leathard, A. (2003) *Interprofessional Collaboration: From Policy to Practice in Health and Social Care*. Hove, Brunner-Routledge.

Lockhart-Wood, K. (2000) 'Collaboration between nurses and doctors in clinical practice', *Journal of Advanced Nursing* 9 (5) pp. 276–80.

Nursing and Midwifery Council (NMC) (2002) *Code of Professional Conduct*. London, NMC.

Nolan, M. (1995) 'Towards an ethos of interdisciplinary practice', *British Medical Journal* 312 (11) pp. 305–6.

Ohlen, J. and Segsten, K. (1998) 'The professional identity of the nurse: concept analysis and development', *Journal of Advanced Nursing* 28 (4) pp. 720–7.

Owens, P., Carrier, J. and Horder, J. (1995) *Interprofessional Issues in Community and Primary Health Care*. Basingstoke, Macmillan Press.

Pirrie, A., Wilson, V., Elsegood, J., Hall, J., Hamilton, S., Harden, R., Lee, D. and Stead, J. (1998) *Evaluating Multidisciplinary Education in Health Care*. Edinburgh, Scottish Council for Research Education.

Porter, S. (1992) 'The poverty of professionalization: a critical analysis of strategies for the occupational advancement of nursing', *Journal of Advanced Nursing* 17 pp. 720–6.

Walby, S., Greenwell, J., Mackay, L. and Soothill, K. (1994) *Medicine and Nursing. Professions in a Changing Health Service*. London, Sage.

Wenger, E., McDermott, R. and Snyder, W. (2002) *Cultivating Communities of Practice*. Boston MA, Harvard Business School Press.

West, M. (2002) 'Sparkling fountains and stagnant ponds: An integrative model of creativity and innovation implementation in work groups', *Applied Psychology: An International Review* 51 pp. 355–87.

West, M., Borrill, C., Dawson, J., Scully, J., Carter, M., Anelay, S., Patterson, M. and Waring, J. (2002) 'The link between the management of employees and patient mortality in acute hospitals', *The International Journal of Human Resource Management* 13 pp. 1299–310.

Wigens, L. (2204) 'Nurses' Management of Individual Caring in Multiple Demand Settings, and the Influence on this of Situated Learning'. Unpublished Ph.D. Thesis. Norwich, University of East Anglia.

9

Becoming an expert caregiver

Lynne Wigens

Learning outcomes

By the end of this chapter you should be able to:

- examine theories regarding the development of care giving expertise;

- develop an understanding of the nature of evidence-based care;

- develop skills in incorporating evidence into practice;

- develop your own ideas about the nature of clinical nursing scholarship;

- understand the potential costs of care.

Introduction

A registered nurse, midwife or health professional, like many health care professionals, works within the guidance of their code of conduct (NMC 2002a). A central theme within this code is the development and maintenance of professional knowledge and competence. This chapter initially addresses the progression of caring skills towards expert practice (Benner 1984) and then moves on to examine the complexity of professional care, arguing that to simply apply research evidence to care situations is inadequate to meet expert working. The chapter closes with a discussion of the potential costs of care.

In lots of situations common sense and opinions are not a good enough basis for making decisions or developing understanding. For example, in deciding which wound dressing to use, the nurse needs knowledge of research studies about wound dressings, the practical skills for the effective application of wound dressings, knowledge about the patient and awareness of the costs of various wound dressing choices. A registered practitioner has a 'responsibility to deliver care based on current evidence, best practice and, where applicable, validated research when it is available' (NMC 2002a section 6.5).

Evidence-based health care involves the 'conscientious, explicit and judicious use of current best evidence about the care of individual patients' (Sackett *et al.* 1996 p. 71). In order to approach care in an evidence-based way a practitioner needs to review the evidence available, thinking carefully and clearly about what makes most sense in influencing their clinical decisions. The best part of the definition means that wherever possible scientific research that is relevant and properly conducted should be used. Evidence-based practice also means integrating individual clinical expertise with the best available external evidence.

Learning to care

Benner (1984) researched how nurses develop from novices to experts, and how they uncover and create knowledge through actual experiences. These experiences occur when an event refines, elaborates or does not confirm former knowledge. Clinical knowledge from this viewpoint is 'a hybrid between naive practical knowledge and unrefined theoretical knowledge' (Benner 1984 p. 8).

Benner used paired interviews with a beginning nurse and an expert nurse who had both been involved in the same situation, and examined the narratives from both participants. An interpretative approach was then used to analyse the data, taking into account the context and the meaning they made of the situation.

Reflective activity

In a similar way to Benner, you could review the thought processes underpinning practice. When you have an opportunity to work alongside an experienced nurse reflect on your understanding of the situation. Then ask them to discuss the incident, taking you through their thought processes. What differences would this have made to the care delivered by the experienced nurse and the care that you would have delivered if you were on your own?

Benner found that the key to expert practice was the ability to experience nursing and then to integrate this into existing and new knowledge. Benner's work (1984) applied the Dreyfus and Dreyfus (1979) model of skill acquisition developed through researching trainee aircraft pilots, which identified five levels of proficiency:

1 novice – shows rigid adherence to taught rules and plans, little situational perception, no discretionary judgement;

2 advanced beginner – needs guidelines for action based on attributes or aspects, situational perceptions still limited, all attributes and aspects treated separately and given equal importance;

3 competent – copes with many forms of information, sees actions partly in terms of long-term goals, conscious planning, standardised and routinised procedures;

4 proficient – sees situations holistically, sees what is most important in a situation, perceives deviations from the normal, decision-making less laboured;

5 expert – not reliant on rules or guidelines, intuitive grasp of situations based on tacit understanding, analytical approaches only used in novel situations or where problems occur, has a vision of what is possible.

Progress within each of these levels relates to three different aspects of skilled performance. These three aspects are: first, development from a reliance on *abstract principles* to the use of *past concrete experiences* as paradigms; second, seeing *each part* of a situation as equally important rather than recognising that only *some parts* are relevant; and third, being an *observer* in the situation rather being *thoroughly engaged*. These aspects have been used within health care educational courses as benchmarks for competencies for assessing individual levels of proficiency at each stage of development.

Benner (1984) also identified seven domains of nursing practice and specific competencies for these:

1 the helping role;
2 the teaching/coaching function;
3 the diagnostic and patient monitoring function ;
4 the effective management of rapidly changing situations;
5 administering and monitoring therapeutic interventions or regimens;
6 monitoring and ensuring the quality of health care practice;
7 organisational and work role competencies.

Benner (1984) recognised a difference between *knowing that* (theoretical knowledge) and *knowing how* (judgement and expertise) (see p. 115), and, as nurses gain experience, their clinical knowledge becomes a blend of practical and theoretical knowledge. Nurses need to maintain their competence and to keep up with a rapidly changing health care environment. Being able to recognise skill levels is a crucial aspect to nurses feeling satisfied in their jobs and staying within nursing.

Learning to care moves practice from a rigid adherence to taught rules to a grasp of the situation that includes tacit context-based understanding of the patient's situation within the context (Benner 1984). For example, the concept of **spirituality** would be handled differently by practitioners working at these different levels of practice. Novice practitioners might ensure that the patient's religious affiliation is assessed on admission as this is an integral component of the admission criteria, but might then not refer to the spiritual dimension of caring in their ongoing practice. Expert caring involves really meeting the spiritual needs of patients. This can be difficult due to the subjectivity of the concept and the different meaning individuals bring to this. There is a risk that it could become an area of neglect as nurses try to avoid the religious/non-religious debate. Spirituality often comes into focus for nurses when their patient/client is facing emotional stress, physical illness or death.

⚷ *Keywords*

Spirituality
A quality that goes beyond religious choice and seeks inspiration, reverence, meaning and purpose.

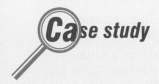

Case study

Read this excerpt from a conversation between a nurse and a patient. What do you pick up from the patient's conversation to indicate her current psychological situation, and how might you carry on this discussion to help meet the patient's spiritual needs?

'I'm sorry about this, I'm making a bit of a fool of myself aren't I. I don't know what's got into me lately. I feel so tired all the time, yet I wake so early . . . I'm snapping at people all the time. God knows what people must think of me.

'I can't seem to cope with work. It's a struggle just getting through the essentials. I just sit there looking like a zombie. At home I just want to shut myself away in a room – away from everything and everybody.

'The worst thing is the panicky feeling I keep getting for no reason. I can't seem to get rid of the feeling that something dreadful is going to happen to me. Sometimes I feel as if I'm going to collapse. I hope you don't mind me talking to you like this, my friend says it's my nerves and I should relax more. It's been a dreadful year one way and another. My father died last year, and my mother manages reasonably well but she's a diabetic and she's having problems with ulcers on her feet. I feel I should have done more for my father when he was ill.

'I feel as if all the enjoyment has gone, and that my son feels I neglect him. I don't know, I don't seem to be much use to anyone when it really matters, I suppose I've just got to sort myself out.'

In deciding on your response you probably thought about how you could help the patient to regain a measure of composure and control over her situation. To help her feel better about the situation you would need to tease out what would assist her, bearing in mind that she needs to make her own decisions. Your response to the quote was probably in the first instance a human one rather than a professional one. However, that response should show an appreciation that involving ourselves at a personal level with the patient's problems and unhappiness could be unhelpful and also that maintaining a professional stance should not suppress natural caring skills.

Expert working calls for excellence in communication, with the ability to develop practitioner–patient relationships and share ideas and information. This also means developing an awareness of the wider context of the patient's family, partners and community. Over time, the relationship deepens as the patient learns to trust in the practitioner. Key concepts important in any relationship include equity, respect, caring, trust, warmth, rapport, being genuine, empathy and acceptance. As in any relationship, the first meeting sets the scene for future communication, and skills such as applying non-verbal reinforcers – e.g. head nods, open questioning and active listening – play a part in starting a caring relationship. Expert nurses modify their care to fit the uniqueness of the patient, and practice at this level requires technical, physical, emotional and intellectual proficiency delivered in a holistic way.

Reflective activity

During your time working in various clinical settings have you seen different forms of nurse–patient relationships? In what ways might patient problems, the length of the patient episode or the age of the patient influence the nurse–patient relationships observed?

When you thought about the relationships you have witnessed in practice you may well have identified a particular practitioner whom you deemed as expert in the way that they developed their practitioner–patient relationship. The intuitive knowing and presence displayed by an expert can be hard for beginning nurses and other health care students to grasp:

> I was invited to watch Mary admit Mrs Wapling for her breast care surgery. Although the questions she was asking and the information she gave was something that Mary did many times that day there was something about the way she did it that showed caring. After this initial meeting Mrs Wapling often asked Mary for support and information. Mary spoke in a calm, clear way, and picked up when Mrs Wapling looked concerned about anything. It would have taken me far longer to get the information, and it only took her about 15 minutes, but at the end she'd found out such a lot about what was worrying Mrs Wapling. I could see the patient's anxiety visibly reducing over the admission/assessment meeting. When I had to admit a patient for breast surgery later on in my placement I tried to copy the way Mary talked to the patient and gained information in a conversational style, rather than just asking questions as they were set out on the assessment tool.
>
> (Student nurse)

Through the process of working alongside experienced nurses, students observe and partially participate in examples of practice where caring values are displayed. Over time students increase the depth of their involvement in the nursing team, and redefine their identity. Novices learn actions, and a holistic explanation, from practitioners in the real world setting. Novices' development occurs through participation in activities beyond their competence with the assistance of skilled professionals who provide the scaffolding for learning. Experts then withdraw as increasing competency is shown by the novice (Rogoff 1990).

Through experience, nurses – like many professionals – rapidly retrieve information from memory about past patient care, and develop standard patterns of problem solving (Simons 2000).

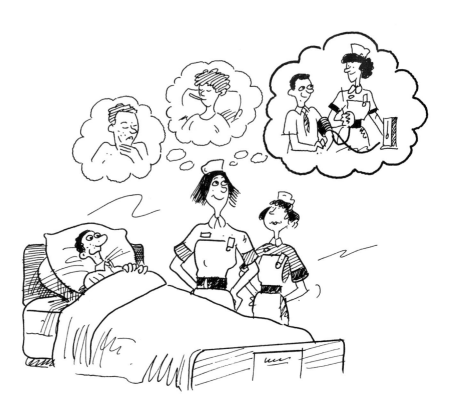

Nursing knowledge acquired in the authentic context has a better chance of being activated when needed in another situation.

People make meaning of a situation based on their past and present learning, which affects how they approach, interpret and make sense of an experience. Learning caring practice requires nurses to celebrate and discuss incidents where caring has made a difference to patient outcomes. The tacit aspects of knowledge that are often the most valuable are shared through storytelling, conversation, coaching and learner support. However, when time is short, decisions are made swiftly and Eraut (1994) believes that this is best understood as a process where there is rapid interpretation of information and decisions made in action. Student nurses may miss out on understanding the mastery behind this swift decision-making.

Nurses are often doing more than one thing at a time, constantly scanning the environment, processing and selecting appropriate data and delivering this to others in the clinical setting, and through this assisting others in the performance of their health care role. These behaviours are often not directly related to the nurse's own immediate working, but they impact on the overall working within the clinical area. An example of this might be the hidden work undertaken by the nurse to arrange a patient discharge from hospital despite organisational constraints such as the limited availability of hospital transport.

Available evidence, the level of complexity and the practitioner's capabilities and disposition are factors that link with the context in affecting decision-making (Eraut 1994). The time available and the complexity of the situation are important variables, and shortages of time force people to adopt a more intuitive approach, and routines that help experienced staff to do things more quickly (Eraut 1994).

Reflective activity

Reflect on an incident where you observed an experienced nurse acting at a high level of practice. What did you particularly notice about their practice?

Would it have been useful to have discussed the situation and questioned them about their decision-making? What stopped you from doing this?

In Priest's (1999) comparison of *expert* and *novice* understanding of psychological care she identified that experts considered information giving as a major aspect, whereas novices placed more emphasis upon their personal qualities. Experts concentrated on handling and working with emotions and novices focusing upon facilitating the expression of emotions, which Priest (1999) suggests is due to the fact that experts are more mindful that encouraging patients to open up emotionally may require time that is unavailable due to competing demands and priorities.

Priest (1999) suggests that specific training programmes in psychological care have not been adopted by nurses, as there is some doubt as to whether this can be taught, whether it is solely developed through experience or indeed whether all nurses can develop psychological care-giving abilities. Nursing students did not expect the theoretical component of nursing courses to contribute anything to their psychological care-giving abilities apart from an insight into psychology. Most nurses expected their psychological care and empathy to develop through trial and error learning, the exposure to practice, and observation of role models and patients, with reflective diaries or portfolios assisting this process.

Senior nurses within a clinical setting play a crucial role in developing the social context for caring work, setting the tone for staff, patients and visitors (Wilson-Barnett *et al.* 1995). Senior nurses are viewed as central to making change happen; they need to be open to new ideas, allow a flexible approach to routines and be supportive to staff so that individualised care can be provided. Lawler (1991) found that expert nurses achieved a fine balance between showing concern and care for the patient while also appearing professional.

Eraut (1994) suggests that there is a close link between client-centredness and continuing to develop one's professional knowledge, as specific individual knowledge needs to be obtained on the spot and delivered through working with colleagues and developing expertise. Used within home and workplace settings, caring as a form of personal knowledge seems far removed from the unique body of research knowledge of traditional professions, but throughout the next sections on advanced practice and evidence-based care, the interrelationships between evidence base and caring skills are explained.

Key points | Top tips

- As nurses move from novice to expert they become able to use many forms of evidence to inform their professional judgements.
- Student nurses can find it difficult to grasp the forms of knowing and presencing displayed by expert nurses, but this is helped by opportunities to work alongside experienced nurses.

Advanced practice

Your nursing practice will change in character over the course of your career and life course, as professional identity becomes fused with your personal sense of identity. Professional identity involves a feeling of being a nurse who can practise with skill and take responsibility for one's own actions, while maintaining an awareness of personal attributes and limitations (Ohlen and Segesten 1998). Leddy and Pepper (1993 p. 75) define professional identity as 'to feel self-certain in her role as a nurse, to feel competent in role experimentation and to clearly articulate their own ideological commitment to the profession'.

The character and form of advanced practice roles within nursing vary across time, context, person, group and institution, and specialisation in nursing has been viewed as essential to the advancement of the profession (Cotton 1997). Within the United Kingdom the debate regarding the need for and effectiveness of specialist nurses continues unabated, and there has been a particular focus on seeking identification of those who operate at a higher level than generalist nurses (NMC 2002b). The changing image of nursing is closely linked to the variable route that specialist roles are now taking in nursing, with some becoming nursing care experts and others appearing to take on medical/medical assistant roles. The boundaries between the work of doctors and that of nurses are changing, with nurses taking over aspects of junior doctors' clinical work (Dowling *et al.* 1995). The aim of these changes is not to produce nurses who practise medicine but to enhance and develop nursing for the benefit of patients. Never before has nursing had the opportunity to progress in this way and create a strong professional identity that is independent of medicine. In doing so, nurses are emerging as confident and competent practitioners able to pioneer new approaches to care.

With the development of these advanced nursing roles there has been a call to ensure standards and competencies are assessed. The United Kingdom Central Council for Nursing, Midwifery and Health Visiting (UKCC) commissioned a project to identify the core competencies for *higher level* nursing practice in 1999. The seven broad headings that were determined were:

- providing effective health care;
- improving quality and health outcomes;
- evaluation and research;
- leading and developing practice;
- innovation and changing practice;
- developing self and others;
- working across professional and organisational boundaries.

It was envisaged that nurses operating at a higher level would collect evidence to indicate their achievements in practice to show their standard of working. This would not require a particular course to evidence this level of practice, but nurses would need to show their learning (NMC 2002b).

Nurses can develop a more positive self-image through career promotion and advanced education (Porter and Porter 1991) and these opportunities are more freely available for those who are willing to take the specialist pathway to career advancement. Post-registration educational programmes are becoming increasingly specialist in nature.

Over to you

Interview an experienced nurse in a senior role, e.g. ward manager, specialist nurse, nurse practitioner, nurse consultant. Find out what informed their career decisions, what courses they have undertaken, and what it is about their role that keeps them motivated to continue their nursing work.

Copp, in her preface to her published study *Facing Impending Death: Experiences of Patients and Their Nurses* (1999), talks of her own movement into the speciality of palliative care in this way:

> In my case, the change from acute to palliative care occurred more by accident than design, motivated more by personal curiosity and a desire to deepen my understanding of the nature of nursing care of the dying. To gain this experience I started work in a local NHS hospice.
>
> (Copp 1999 p. vi)

Clinical scholars are viewed as having high levels of curiosity, critical thinking, continuous learning, reflection and the ability to seek and use a spectrum of resources/evidence to improve clinical interventions. Clinical scholarship requires a willingness to scrutinise practice, challenging the theories and practice that have already been learnt and looking for better ways of doing things. Clinical scholarship will not always be the product of maturity, as even though experience is important, many years in practice can still lead to doing things the way they have always been done.

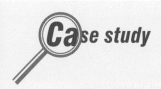

Case study

Nichole, a new tissue viability nurse specialist, had several years of experience as a senior staff nurse, preceptor and mentor within both surgical and community settings. She identified quite early on in her new role that pressure sore prevention was a crucial area for improvement within the hospital. She started by working with link nurses and others in documenting the baseline incidence and prevalence of hospital acquired pressure sores. The team then used their findings, combined with a comprehensive literature review, to design care protocols for the prevention and treatment of pressure sores. This included the use of a validated assessment tool and an algorithm to aid in determining care decisions. A further step in the change process involved Nichole and her team evaluating the supplies and devices used for pressure sore care from a range of perspectives, including the research base, ease of use and cost-effectiveness. She then negotiated with suppliers through a tendering process to achieve cost benefits within this change in practice, and she encouraged, through clinical leadership, the different ward areas to benchmark their new practice comparing the effectiveness of their implementation of the practice change to other ward areas. As well as delivering in-house study events to disseminate the new pressure sore practices, Nichole also worked with the local educational institute to develop a post-registration module for staff nurses that would be a useful introduction to the subject for link nurses. A year later the original prevalence and incidence data collection was replicated and indicated a significant improvement within the NHS Trust. The team celebrated these results by sharing their information through a range of mediums at a local (newsletter) and national (conferences/articles) level. This all took a lot of time and commitment.

Do you think Nichole is displaying clinical scholarship?

Can you identify the following stages in this change in practice?

- observing
- synthesising
- analysing
- disseminating

Clinical scholarship is value based, and appreciating your own values as a health care practitioner plays an important part in informing your care. Nurses are viewed as caring about their work and this is grounded in professional values (Thompson *et al.* 2001). Whatever your values, there is a requirement that they do not influence patient care detrimentally. The first step to ensuring this involves exploring your own value base.

Over to you

In this activity a number of value statements are given. Decide whether these are things that you value, do not mind, or do not particularly value:

- to die in my own home;
- to be able to refuse treatment;
- to get advice from others on diet and exercise;
- to realise that my partner is having an affair with someone;
- to be told the truth on request;
- to have an understanding GP;
- to be offered a new, relatively untested drug;
- to be in surroundings that are familiar to me;
- to be able to maintain the living standard I normally have;
- to be able to maintain my appearance;
- to go on holiday.

The things that you valued within the exercise are often some of the potential issues that patients that you care for have to deal with. Although individual responses and values are different, this exercise was presented here to give you some insight into appreciating individual differences, and how values affect patient expectations of caregivers.

Autonomy is also important within clinical scholarship. It is not just about having a sense of independence within practice; it is about a sense of ownership and leadership within one's work, and being accountable for the outcomes. Clinical scholarship is also about creativity in thinking, allowing students to challenge decisions, and not waiting for management to sort out problems.

New nursing roles are constantly changing and expanding, creating new opportunities for value-based, autonomous and creative practice. Nurses need to be able to solve problems, to develop solutions that may include creating new nursing roles, and to carry them out. To do this effectively nurses are acknowledging the importance of a clinical evidence and research base to guide practice.

- A nurse's professional identity involves skilled practice, taking responsibility for actions and feeling competent in role experimentation.
- New expert roles within nursing are constantly emerging and being implemented.
- Professional values, autonomy and creativity of practice underpin clinical scholarship.

Evidence-based practice

The earliest use of the term *evidence-based nursing* within nursing journals was in the early 1990s, and the term is commonly an umbrella term for information management, clinical judgement, professional development and managed care (French 2002). Even though the use of this term has only come to the fore in the past decade, evidence-based nursing is increasingly replacing the term *research-based nursing*. The word *evidence* in this concept tends to relate to primary research findings, and shows a shift in health care provision away from basing decisions on past practice and opinion. The need to integrate best available external evidence with individual clinical expertise is also included.

Evidence-based practice involves a process beginning with knowing what clinical questions to ask. First, an area of practice is identified for which the evidence base is not known. Then the practitioner needs to search for relevant literature using a range of sources, e.g. library, electronic databases on the Internet and colleagues. If systematic reviews (summaries of all the available research in an area) already exist, these should be used. If a systematic review is not available the next step is to 'grade' or determine the strength of the research. The strength of evidence on which to base a clinical decision varies from topic to topic. Within evidence-based practice, types of evidence are seen as relative with certain forms being viewed as stronger evidence. The Cochrane Collaboration is a body that has been set up to commission and produce reviews of research evidence. The library of systematic reviews produced help practitioners to access research evidence, and this should reduce variability in health care. The grading of evidence usually follows this form:

1 systematic review of a series of randomised controlled trials;
2 one well-designed randomised controlled trial;
3 at least one well-designed cohort study (non-random);

4 well-designed non-experimental studies;

5 expert opinion based on clinical evidence or descriptive studies.

The highest level or strongest evidence (1) is obtained from randomised controlled trials (RCTs) and involves an experimental design comparing the outcomes between two or more groups randomly assigned to a treatment/intervention group versus another strategy/no treatment/intervention group. To minimise distortion in the results of the research, neither researchers nor patients know which group is receiving the treatment/intervention being examined. This is sometimes referred to as *blinding*. Within the hierarchy of evidence RCTs are regarded as the gold standard evidence base as they are able to produce the strongest research evidence. The next level of evidence includes experiments without randomisation, such as the study of one cohort/group of patients. Non-experimental research is placed lower in the hierarchy of research evidence, with expert opinions being viewed as the lowest level of evidence upon which to base clinical decisions.

Once all the relevant literature has been read and critically examined, the practitioner should then share this information with other staff, finding out whether they think it is relevant to practice in their setting. A comparison needs to be made between the best practice identified through the literature search and the practice that currently exists. The question then needs to be asked as to whether a change in practice is needed. The evidence found may support current practice, or there may be a need to change practice. The next stage will be to implement the findings of the evidence-based practice review within the clinical area. This may involve translating the evidence into a useful, usable and relevant package and in a form that suits the area of health care work. It involves combining research evidence with ethical, organisational and other expert advice in an easily accessible format that all practitioners can use within the practice setting, for example a **clinical guideline**.

Old habits can be hard to break, so there is a need to maintain the change in practice over a reasonable time period. Practice developments should incorporate ways of demonstrating effectiveness, and the criteria for evaluating the impact of the intervention must be identified and agreed before implementing any change. This has to be done scientifically and involves the rigorous collection of baseline information on current practice, followed by ongoing evaluation against clear outcomes after the change has taken place. The final aspect of the evidence-based practice process is the collation of evaluations or assessments identifying the impact of practice changes. This is often undertaken through an audit. Clinical audit provides a means by which judgements can be made

⊶ᴛ *Keywords*

Clinical guideline

A written record, systematically developed and designed from best evidence, which offers guidance or recommendations for practice in a given situation.

against predetermined standards based on clinical guidelines. Ongoing practice development is then supported by continuous application of the audit cycle involving standard setting, observation of practice, evaluation against standards, action and constant review.

Understanding the stages of implementing evidence-based practice is not all that is required for effective evidence-based practice to occur. Health care professionals also need leadership and support from their organisation, appraisal skills to identify the potential risks and benefits involved in implementing changes, and the skills of critiquing research.

The suggested hierarchy of levels of evidence places RCTs at the top of the hierarchy, and experiential or clinical judgement at the bottom, but Rolfe (2002) argues that power is sited with the scientific researcher and denied to the nurse. The conformity and standardisation inherent in evidence-based practice can lead to the devaluing of practice knowledge. The integration of qualitative or interpretative research into evidence-based practice is also not straightforward as interpretation is often undertaken from a traditional research stance, even though particular areas of nursing, such as communication and relationship development with patients, seem to be best served through qualitative and interpretative research.

✍ *Over to you*

Nursing models are difficult to validate through traditional research methods. Take a look at the following journal article: Erci, B. *et al.* (2003) 'Issues and innovations in nursing practice. The effectiveness of Watson's Caring Model on the quality of life and blood pressure of patients with hypertension', *Journal of Advanced Nursing* 41 (2) pp. 130–9.

This study involved 52 patients with hypertension in four health care units in Turkey. Patients were given demographic questionnaires, filled in information on a quality of life scale, and had their blood pressure measured. The nurses received training in Watson's ten carative processes.

An adapted version of Watson's ten key carative processes within nursing are listed here:

1 delivering practice within a humanistic/altruistic and loving context;

2 being authentically present, instilling faith and hope;

3 cultivating sensitivity to self and to others;

4 developing and sustaining a helping/trusting relationship;

5 being supportive of the expression of positive and negative feelings;

6 using self creatively, and all ways of knowing, as part of the caring process;

7 engaging in genuine teaching/learning experiences;

> 8 creating a healing environment (physical/psychological/social), including dignity and respect;
>
> 9 assisting with basic needs;
>
> 10 attending to the spiritual dimensions of life and death.
>
> The nurses visited the patients once a week for three months (measuring their blood pressure on each occasion). The researchers found statistically significant differences between the pre-intervention and post-intervention scores for general well-being, physical symptoms and activity and medical interaction.
>
> Now that you have looked at the Erci *et al.* article, what are your views about this type of research method being used to research this nursing model?

There is a fear of a cookbook approach to clinical practice, as the judging of which research evidence to use has often already been done for the nurses (Walsh and Wigens 2003). Generic protocols are in some instances being applied ritualistically, and the individuality of patients and the uniqueness of different contexts can be overlooked:

> Nurses no longer need to choose which papers to read, to assess them for themselves, and to engage in debate over their strengths and weakness. Indeed, they do not need to read original pages at all, merely to digest summaries of papers selected for them as being 'best'.
>
> (Rolfe 2002 p. 10)

Nurses working in demanding practice settings can see reference to evidence sources as a low priority. Research evidence is only one form of knowledge for health care workers to use to make judgements about what to do in an endless variety of situations that affect their clinical practice (Walsh and Wigens 2003). The perceived dominance of scientific or empirical knowledge within evidence-based practice creates a difficulty for nurses, who utilise a range of forms of knowledge in a context-specific approach within their everyday practice.

Within nursing there has been a long-standing disagreement between those who emphasise the technical and scientific aspects of nursing, and those who highlight its caring aspects. Bostrom and Suter (1993) found that only 23 per cent (n=1588) of the nurses they surveyed believed they had made a research-based practice change during their career. Research-based systematic studies were seen as more useful for nurses than single studies, but library and electronic resources were almost exclusively used when undertaking academic courses for continuous professional development or developing a protocol or standard. Practitioners considered much of the research generated as asking irrelevant questions, lacking generalisation, and as having unrealistic resource implications.

Text-based and electronic sources of research-based information are perceived as limited in their usefulness for nurses, as human sources – clinically trusted and credible individuals – are overwhelmingly perceived as the most useful in reducing the uncertainties of nursing decisions (Thompson *et al.* 2001). Clinical credibility is necessary for perceiving a source of evidence as useful; for instance, the specialist clinical advice given by clinical nurse specialists who stockpile information on their subject – and by their associated link nurses – is seen as credible (Thompson *et al.* 2001).

Even though guidance is derived from others, it should not be assumed that this has no basis in research knowledge because 'it is clinical experience – either one's own or that of others (including patients) – that is afforded the highest weighting in clinical decision-making' (Thompson *et al.* 2001 p. 382).

The knowledge developed by individual nurses through their decision-making and experience differs from formal scientific knowledge that is published in books. To give an example, in performing a urinary catheterisation the inexperienced nurse may rely on knowledge gained from physiology texts that provide diagrams showing genitalia. Experienced nurses will know that it is not unusual for people's genitalia to differ and that in some instances the urethra may not be sited in the immediately expected location. Such nurses also know that they need to value this type of information and pass this on to less experienced colleagues (Eraut 1994), but may be too busy to do much about it in any structured way. Benner *et al.* (1996) found that experienced nurses tend to pass on this type of knowledge through informal processes such as storytelling. Storytelling is both an art form, in which events can be recounted and interpreted, and a process of negotiation, with the listener providing something that is either entertaining, educational, meaningful or participatory (Livo and Rietz 1986; Sandelowski 1996). In nursing, storytelling is a vehicle for pooling expertise, for example by creating warnings to others about particular situations that are more easily memorised than formal procedures or rules. Alternatively, storytelling may help practitioners to interpret events, integrate new perceptions and understandings with established collective knowledge and explore possible new scenarios. In so doing, nurses create a vocabulary of precedents for dealing with clinical situations (Benner *et al.* 1996; Sandelowski 1996; Shearing and Erickson 1991).

Professional practice is more complex than simply applying theory to practice, since it involves a professional juggling of situational demands, intuition, experiences and knowledge (Schön 1991). Practitioners do not apply research findings in a simple deductive process; they need time to think, translate and relate the research findings to their particular setting. Successful implementation of evidence-based practice occurs when the evidence is robust, the context is receptive to change and there is appropriate monitoring, strong leadership and facilitation of the change (Harvey *et al.* 2002). Timing is important to the perception of relevance and to professional involvement and engagement with research. The extent to which a given piece of evidence is utilised by an individual in practice depends on their sense of the situation and this inevitably involves professional judgement.

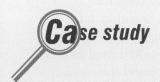

Case study

Mrs Green is a 78-year old woman who has a history of chronic venous leg ulcers and heart disease. She lives alone at home, has several cats and rarely leaves her house. She spends most of her day sitting in an armchair in her front room watching the television. She can move to the toilet when she needs it, but the house is cluttered and difficult to move around in. She has been admitted and discharged from hospital on a number of occasions. Although her leg ulcers have been diagnosed as venous in origin she has not wanted to have compression therapy (the treatment of choice to heal venous ulcers – see Cullum *et al.* 1998).

She often removes the dressings soon after the community nurse visits, and cat hair is regularly found in the wounds.

You would expect wound management practice to be based on the best possible evidence. However, in this situation organisational and professional beliefs are different to the patient's beliefs. Mrs Green could be viewed as non-compliant or 'difficult'.

What might be your next steps if you were the community nurse in this situation?

The fact that nurses use evidence in a way that is context-sensitive, and call on a range of knowledge in practice, does not mean that nurses perceive research as unimportant. McSherry's (1997) survey found that 95 per cent of the nurses interviewed (n=765) stated that nursing research played an important role in improving patient care, even though they were largely unable to explain this within their own practice. This would suggest that a positive attitude towards research does not automatically imply research utilisation. Barriers to research utilisation include: the absence of support within the clinical setting; lack of access and ability to critique research; a lack of consensus within the body of research on a particular aspect of practice; poor quality research; and lack of relevant research. When referring to health care interventions overall, Baker (1996) estimates that only about 15 per cent of health care is research based. He goes on to suggest that at best this will only increase to around 50 per cent, so any idea that nursing could become wholly research based is really unrealistic.

Busy health care professionals want to use research but can find it difficult to find the time to keep abreast of advances in practice through reading journals and other external evidence, let alone undertaking their own research studies. There are, however, advantages for health care professionals who practise in an evidence-based way, as it means that their knowledge base continues to improve and that they have increased confidence in their clinical decision-making.

Within the NHS change is a way of life, and the interest in evidence-based practice has led to questions about the ways to influence clinical practice. Implementing change is possible, but it is a complex business that takes time, resources and stamina.

The important issues are to know the current situation, build on what is already working, use a range of approaches and use good project management techniques. Clinical audit is often used as a way of analysing the gap between current practice and the research evidence. The next step involves assessing the attitudes of people who will need to change their current working and any resource consequences. People cannot change unless they have the space and time to absorb and understand the evidence, so just circulating information in a busy clinical context will not lead to change. Wherever possible, existing communication systems should be used to disseminate progress and updates. The leadership of the practice change needs to be someone who has a reputation and position within the organisation and has project management skills.

Key points | **Top tips**

The trick in making an evidence-based practice change is to make best use of what is known already and to focus implementation initiatives on topics that have a robust evidence base. You need to believe that change is possible, although it might be difficult.

Avoid the following traps:

- spending too much time looking for evidence;
- involving the wrong people;
- ignoring the impact on the service;
- keeping others in the dark;
- leaving patients out of the discussion;
- assuming that staff will turn up to training sessions;
- creating glossy guidelines.

> **Key points** Top tips
>
> - Evidence-based practice has become increasingly important in health care, and research in nursing is becoming more available.
> - Evidence should be critiqued and evaluated before decisions are made to change practice.
> - It is probably unrealistic to expect all nursing practice to be underpinned by research as scientific evidence cannot always be used to support complex professional practice.

Potential costs of care

The generalist nature of nursing means that its value is poorly recognised with regard to patient/health care outcomes, even though nurses deliver 80 per cent of direct patient care (Antrobus 1997). Benner and Wrubel (1989) define caring as combining thoughts, feelings and actions, and being connected and concerned towards the patient. It is suggested that the nature of caring and clinical judgement is intangible, and hence devalued and invisible (Benner and Wrubel 1989), and that the technical competencies required in health care sometimes make it difficult to foster caring relationships. Benner (1984) points out that so much is lost when caring is not recorded, and, without knowing where we are, it will be difficult to make provision for development in the future. Nursing behaviours that minimise nursing work as 'women's work' and naturally inherent, rather than learnt through practice, can create tensions within the profession because 'as long as society overvalues technology's heroic promises . . . and fails to recognise the care required to support such a technological self-understanding, those who provide care will feel the stress of being invisible and undervalued by society' (Benner and Wrubel 1989 p. 398).

In Smith's (1992) exploration of student nurses' socialisation processes, students were found to experience anxiety and stress because their emotional labour (previously discussed in Chapter 1) was largely unrecognised and undervalued, and their workloads meant that there was only time to meet the physical and technical needs of patients. The little things of caring were not being recognised or costed in the work process. Nurses wanted to work with people but worked in an organisational environment that placed emphasis on getting the work done and rewarded non-patient-oriented activities (Smith 1992).

The concept of emotional labour has helped in understanding how emotions have become a commodity in the work environment, just like technical skills such as prescribing. However, it is still difficult to measure the effects of caring within a health system where budgets are tight and targets often relate to efficiency. There are costs to emotional labour for individual employees, as the function of the emotions is to represent in a conscious and consistent way, through distinctive feelings and thoughts, the personally significant aspects of situations. It is suggested that managing emotional labour can cause nurses to lose the personal aspects, and signalling function, of emotions.

There are costs to individual employees in terms of the amount of emotional labour they provide and the psychological and emotional energy that labour consumes. It is suggested that managing emotional labour requires nurses to place others before themselves to an extent that aspects of their own beings become neglected or even damaged because 'in dividing our sense of self, in order to save the "real" self from unwelcome intrusions, we necessarily relinquish a healthy sense of wholeness' (Hochschild 1983 p. 183).

The costs to the worker of emotional labour can include burnout, guilt, blame for being insincere and cynicism at recognising when they are acting. Different levels of illness and disability create differing demands for nursing care, and the levels of nurses caring can be depleted through physical and/or emotional exhaustion (Benner and Wrubel 1989). Ultimately this may lead to nurses leaving their employment and the profession.

James (1992) suggests that in practice individualised care may only amount to finding out enough about patients to know when to interrupt routines to attend to individual requirements. Even when there has been robust evidence available for many years to support a change in practice – e.g. the reduced amount of pre-operative fasting time required for patients having a general anaesthetic – this is sometimes not implemented. Nursing teams can still be found stopping diet and fluids at the same time for all patients on a morning surgical list, meaning that some patients have to fast for too long and risk dehydration and electrolyte imbalance. The ritual task of nil by mouth takes precedence in these nursing teams for a number of reasons:

- To individualise the time of fasting on a surgical ward is perceived as creating more work.
- They fear the complications associated with the aspiration of the stomach contents.
- They have discounted the role of the patient in taking responsibility for their own individualised fasting.

- They fear repercussions if the patient's pre-operative fasting is missed and surgery delayed.

Allen (2000) found that, although nurses were supportive of the principle of involving patients, family and friends in care, implementing this in practice placed additional demands on their limited time and undermined the ability to control their work. When the management of nursing care operates on the industrial basis of an assembly line, personal service is much harder to deliver (Hochschild 1983).

Over to you

Read the following excerpt from a discussion with a nurse working in a day surgery unit. Do you think she is discussing emotional labour?

'I always find that if a patient says "Oh it's a bit like a conveyor belt here" I always feel as if we've failed a bit somehow. It's very difficult to disguise that you've got a lot of patients . . . and very quick procedures so it does seem in and out. If you're a patient in the bay with three or four others and if we haven't got all the beds, and we've got to make the bed again for the next one coming in, you can't really disguise that fact, but we do our best.'

(Wigens 1997)

Institutional incentives to care do not explicitly exist within current NHS working. However, within the NHS the debate about how quality of care is to be measured appears to have increased in proportion to the rising pressure for resources (Attree 2001). Measures of care can relate to:

- resources for care, including having enough staff and the right skill mix, the right equipment and adequate finances to deliver quality care;
- the care processes of assessment, planning, implementing and evaluating care that adhere to best practice standards;
- the communication and organisation of care;
- humanistic or caring qualities of practitioners;
- meeting patients' care needs and final outcomes.

If nurses are to start to cost caring and changes in health care, they may want to consider collecting evidence of quality of care using tools that contain criteria that examine a range of these quality dimensions. It is much easier to predict the costs of a new piece of technical equipment than to assess the financial value of caring, but caring behaviours should be included in any cost versus benefit analysis of managed health care. Caring interventions such as support, education and communication, like evidence-based practice, impact on health care outcomes and should therefore be considered in developing health care services.

Key points Top tips

- The caring aspects of practice are often not recognised within health care management.
- The multiple demands placed on nurses can lead to burnout and exhaustion, and affect the retention of nurses in clinical settings.
- There is a need to measure care explicitly in a range of ways, and to cost this into any change in practice.

Conclusion

Evidence exists to inform and guide practice rather than dictate it. What constitutes good evidence is the subject of continual debate, and the best evidence can in certain situations be justifiably ignored. An expert nurse may decide to ignore research and this may be based on another form of evidence or knowing, such as ethics. Within this chapter the need for nurses to draw on evidence from different sources has been examined. It has been argued that caring requires more than just the 'scientific' grading of evidence. Science and art are both important in effective nursing care. The evidence from interpersonal relationships and patient involvement can be strong factors in determining best practice. Research needs to be relevant to the clinical situation, acceptable to the professional and the patient, comprehensive, accurate, easily accessible and understandable if nurses and other health care professionals are to implement the findings. Patients often experience stressful life events, and they benefit from the comfort and support that instrumental caring (that is to say, what the carer does) and expressive caring (the way that the care is delivered) combined can provide. Being able to deliver care that is supported by current evidence and valued within their organisation can provide nurses with a sense of satisfaction in their work and the motivation to continue improving their practice.

Rapid recap

1 What are the seven domains of nursing identified by Benner?
2 Identify some ways that students can learn from expert nurses.
3 Define the term clinical scholarship.
4 What is evidence-based practice?
5 List and outline barriers to the implementation of evidence-based practice.

References

Allen, D. (2000) 'Negotiating the role of expert carers on an adult hospital ward', *Sociology of Health and Illness* 22 (2) pp. 149–71.

Antrobus, S. (1997) 'An analysis of nursing in context: the effects of current health policy', *Journal of Advanced Nursing* 21 pp. 172–83.

Attree, M. (2001) 'A study of the criteria used by healthcare professionals, managers and patients to represent and evaluate quality care', *Journal of Nursing Management* 9 pp. 67–78.

Baker, M. (1996) 'Developing, disseminating and using research information, in M. Baker and S. Kirk (eds) *Research and Development for the NHS*. London, National Association for Health Authorities and Trusts.

Benner, P. (1984) *From Novice to Expert: Excellence and Power in Clinical Nursing Practice*. Menlo Park CA, Addison-Wesley.

Benner, P. and Wrubel, J. (1989) *The Primacy of Caring: Stress and Coping in Health and Illness*. Berkeley CA, Addison-Wesley.

Benner, P., Tanner, C. and Chesla, C. (1996) *Expertise in Nursing Practice. Caring, Clinical Judgement and Ethics*. New York, Springer Publishing Company.

Bostrom, J. and Suter, W. (1993) 'Research utilisation. Making the link to practice', *Journal of Nursing Staff Development* 9, pp. 28–34.

Copp, G. (1999) *Facing Impending Death: Experiences of Patients and Their Nurses*. London, Nursing Times Books.

Cotton, A. (1997) 'Power, knowledge, and the discourse of specialization in nursing', *Clinical Nurse Specialist* 11 (1) 25–9.

Cullum, N., Fletcher, A., Nelson, E. and Sheldon, T. (1998) 'Compression bandages and stockings in the treatment of venous leg ulcers', The Cochrane Library 4. Oxford, Update Software Ltd.

Dowling, S., Barrett, S., and West, R. (1995) 'With nurse practitioners, who needs house officers?', *British Medical Journal* 311 (7000) pp. 309–13.

Dreyfus, H. and Dreyfus, S. (1979) *The Scope, Limits and Training Implications of Three Models of Aircraft Pilot Emergency Response Behaviour.* Unpublished Report, USAF Grant AFOSR-78-3594, University of California, Berkeley.

Dreyfus, H. and Dreyfus, S. (1986) *Mind over Machine: The Power of Human Intuition and Expertise in the Era of the Computer*. New York, The Free Press.

Eraut, M. (1994) (4th edition, 1999) Developing *Professional Knowledge and Competence*. Lewes, Falmer Press.

Erci, B., Sayan, A., Kiliç, D., Sahin, O. and Güngörmüs, Z. (2003) 'Issues and innovations in nursing practice. The effectiveness of Watson's Caring Model on the quality of life and blood pressure of patients with hypertension', *Journal of Advanced Nursing* 41 (2) pp. 130–9.

French, P. (2002) 'What is the evidence on evidence-based nursing? An epistemological concern', *Journal of Advanced Nursing* 37 (3) pp. 250–7.

Harvey, G., Loftus-Hills, A., Rycroft-Malone, J., Titchen, A., Kitson, A., McCormack, B. and Seers, K. (2002) 'Getting evidence into practice: the role and function of facilitation', *Journal of Advanced Nursing* 37 (6) pp. 577–88.

Hochschild A (1983) *The Managed Heart. Commercialisation of Human Feeling*. Berkeley CA, University of California Press.

James, N. (1992) 'Care = organisation + physical labour + emotional labour', *Sociology of Health and Illness* 14 pp. 488–509.

Kilkus, S. (1993) 'Assertiveness amongst professional nurses', *Journal of Advanced Nursing* 18 pp. 1324–30.

Lawler, L. (1991) *Behind the Screens: Nursing, Somology, and the Problem of the Body*. Melbourne, Churchill Livingstone.

Leddy, S. and Pepper, J. (1993) *Conceptual Bases for Professional Nursing*, 3rd edn. Philadelphia PA, Lippincott.

Livo, N. and Rietz, S. (1986) *Storytelling. Process and Practice*. Littleton, CO, Libraries Ltd Inc.

McSherry, R. (1997) 'What do registered nurse and midwives feel and know about research?', *Journal of Advanced Nursing* 25 (5) pp. 985–98.

Nursing and Midwifery Council (NMC) (2002a) *Code of Professional Conduct*. London, NMC.

Nursing and Midwifery Council (NMC) (2002b) *UKCC Report of the Higher Level of Practice Pilot Project*. London, MNC.

Ohlen, J. and Segesten, K. (1998) 'The professional identity of the nurse: concept analysis and development', *Journal of Advanced Nursing* 28 (4) pp. 720–7.

Porter, R. and Porter, M. (1991) 'Career development: our professional responsibility', *Journal of Professional Nursing* 7 pp. 208–12.

Priest, H. (1999) 'Novice and expert perceptions of psychological care and the development of psychological caregiving abilities', *Nurse Education Today* 19 pp. 556–63.

Rogoff, B. (1990) *Apprenticeship in Thinking*. New York, Oxford University Press.

Rolfe, G. (2002) 'Faking a difference: evidence based nursing and the illusion of diversity', *Nurse Education Today* 22 pp. 3–12.

Sackett, D., Rosenburg, W., Muir Gray, J., Haynes, R. and Richardson, W. (1996) 'Evidence-based medicine: what it is and what it isn't', *British Medical Journal* 312 pp. 71–2.

Sandelowski, M. (1996) 'Truth/storytelling in nursing inquiry', Chapter 9 in J. Kikuchi, H. Simmons and D. Romyn (eds) *Truth in Nursing Inquiry*. Thousand Oaks CA, Sage.

Schön, D. (1991) *The Reflective Turn: Case Studies in Educational Practice*. New York, Teachers Press.

Shearing, C. and Ericson, R. (1991) 'Culture as figurative action', *British Journal of Sociology* 42 (4) pp. 481–586.

Simons, H. (2000) *On What Evidence Do We Act in Developing and Using Professional Knowledge?* Keynote Paper: Reinterpreting Evidence Based Practice: A Narrative Approach. London, A collaborative Action Research Network Conference.

Smith, P. (1992) *The Emotional Labour of Nursing. How Nurses Care*. London, Macmillan.

Thompson, C., McCaughan, D., Cullum, N., Shelden, T., Mulhall, A. and Thompson, D. (2001) 'Research information in nurses' clinical decision-making: What is useful?', *Journal of Advanced Nursing* 36 (3) pp. 376–88.

Walsh, M. and Wigens, L. (2003) *Introduction to Research*. Cheltenham, Nelson Thornes.

Watson, J. (1996) 'Watson's theory of transpersonal caring', in P. Walker and B. Neuman (eds) *Blueprint for Use of Nursing Models: Education, Research, Practice and Administration*. New York, NLN Press, pp. 141–84.

Wigens, L. (1997) 'The conflict between "new nursing" and "scientific management" as perceived by surgical nurses', *Journal of Advanced Nursing* 25 (6) pp. 1116–22.

Wilson-Barnett, J., Butterworth, T., White, E., Twinn, S., Davies, S. and Riley, L. (1995) 'Clinical support and the Project 2000 nursing student: factors influencing this process', *Journal of Advanced Nursing* 21 pp. 1152–8.

10

Health policies and care

Jayne Holmes

Learning outcomes

By the end of this chapter you should be able to:

- appreciate the way health policy influences approaches to care;

- recognise the aims of the NHS plan and their implications for nursing care;

- understand the concept of clinical governance;

- recognise the importance of standard setting for nursing care;

- understand the application of benchmarking and its contribution to improving the quality of nursing care;

- recognise the implications of patient and public involvement in health care.

Introduction

Current health policy is directed towards reform of the health service to meet the health care needs of patients in the twenty-first century. These policies represent the most radical overhaul of the National Health Service since it began in 1948. Inherent in these reforms is the recognition that both health care knowledge and practice have developed considerably since the Second World War and will continue to do so. In addition, societal and demographic changes have created a more diverse society with quite differing expectations to those that pertained when the health service was first set up. In those days access to medical treatment was a luxury that many could not afford. A health service that was free at the point of delivery was an extraordinary concept intended to improve the health of the nation, whereas now it is regarded as a taken-for-granted part of everyday life. Since the 1940s, our understanding of health has increased tremendously and we have come to understand that simply providing a service is not enough. We now have to be concerned also about the nature and standard of that service and ensure that it responds to changing needs. Such needs are evident when we consider the nature and effects of health inequalities that may be due to factors such as poverty, social exclusion, work or the area in which people live. Such inequalities may be compounded by lack of access to appropriate services or poor standards of treatment or care.

Inevitably, the complexity and diversity of modern health care is reflected in current health policy, as is the need for reform in order to provide the best standard of treatment and care for everyone in a consistent way throughout the UK. This chapter helps you to develop an understanding of this policy with reference to your own field of practice. It begins with an explanation of the context in which the need for change has arisen and then presents an overview of the reforms introduced through the NHS Plan (DOH 2000).

Various aspects of these reforms are then discussed in detail. These include the National Institute for Clinical Excellence, National Service Frameworks and clinical governance. The chapter closes with a discussion of the changing role of patients and the general public in terms of their involvement in all aspects of service planning and delivery.

Background to recent health policy

It is difficult to examine recent health policies and their impact on care without briefly understanding the context in which they were developed. Therefore, a brief consideration of health policy from a historical perspective is outlined here.

It is generally accepted that the NHS is a victim of its own success, in that, since its inception in 1948, people are living healthier as well as longer lives (DOH 2000). However, this – along with developing medical and technological knowledge – is placing increasing demands on an already over-stretched system. Successive governments have tried to address these issues by introducing policies and reforms designed to make the NHS more efficient and effective, with only partial success.

Looking back over only the last 15 years, there have been major changes in health policy that have sought to ensure the efficient and effective use of resources as demands on the health service have increased and increases in funding have not been available on the scale needed. Reforms of the Health Service in 1990 and the following years introduced the concept of the internal market with the separation of responsibility for purchasing and responsibility for providing health care. The government at the time felt that efficiency and effectiveness would be increased if competition was introduced and providers of health care functioned as businesses. Purchasers would have a choice of providers and therefore be able to obtain best value for money, and care would improve as hospitals competed to obtain contracts for the provision of services in order to survive.

However, negative consequences of such competition soon emerged, and the internal market was seen as divisive. There was inequity of service provision and a reluctance to share developments. Thus, in 1997, the newly elected Labour government sought to dismantle the internal market (DOH 1997), while retaining the principles of improving efficiency, promoting excellence and increasing access to services.

A ten-year programme of modernisation for the NHS introduced a number of different approaches to make the NHS more responsive to the needs and expectations of the government and the public. These included national standards for the delivery of care, thus removing the postcode lottery, whereby access – and in many cases approaches – to treatment varied according to where in the country the patient lived. The aim was to ensure equity of access to high-quality care for all patients. In doing so the Labour government hoped to rebuild public confidence in the NHS.

Partnership working was to be encouraged by the introduction of local *Primary Care Groups*, which would eventually be responsible for the commissioning of services. The establishment of these groups with the freedom to make decisions on how best to use their resources within the framework of their *Health Improvement Programme* was a significant step towards a primary care-led NHS. It provided clear incentives to move as much health care as possible into the community, thus reducing the use of hospital services (Ham 2004). It also encouraged staff within primary care, especially those with day-to-day patient contact, to influence the provision of care and prioritise the allocation of resources.

Reflective activity

From the end of the 1980s health policies have emphasised the involvement of clinical staff in management. With this comes the management of resources.

Consider the advantages and disadvantages of this for the staff and the health service.

What ethical issues might this create for staff?

The NHS Plan

The reforms launched in 1997 were intended to be phased in over a period of ten years but two years later, and despite increased funding, the NHS experienced increasing pressures on its services and there were difficulties in achieving the access targets, which resulted in widespread negative publicity. In response, a new and comprehensive set of reforms were launched (DOH 2000). The NHS Plan made a commitment to increase capacity by the allocation of additional resources. In addition, it addressed many of the issues of particular concern to patients:

- investment in NHS staff: including more consultants, GPs, nurses and therapists, a new pay system, provision of on-site nurseries and improvements in the working environment;
- changed systems: including the establishment of a modernisation agency to support improvement, core national standards and targets, and devolved responsibility for high-performing Trusts;
- development of partnership working between health and social care services;
- changes for NHS doctors: including increases in training posts and new contracts for GPs and consultants;
- changes for nurses, midwives, therapists and other NHS staff: new and expanded roles for nurses, introduction of 'modern matrons', individual learning accounts for support staff and a focus on leadership;
- changes for patients: with greater patient choice, increased availability of patient information, a Patient Advice and Liaison Service available in every Trust, revised consent procedures, greater patient representation throughout the NHS, Patient and Public Involvement Forums, and scrutiny by local authorities;
- reduced waiting times for treatment: with specific targets for outpatient appointments, GP appointments, elective surgery and A&E;
- health improvement: reducing inequalities by the provision of increased resources to deprived areas, new screening programmes and interventions to improve the health of children;
- clinical priorities: cancer, coronary heart disease and mental health;
- older people's services: promoting dignity, security and independence, improving access to services, and reviews of funding systems.

(DOH 2000)

The NHS Plan placed nurses at the centre of the NHS reforms and provided exciting opportunities for the profession (DOH 2000). Nurses provide a large percentage of the care and treatment for each individual patient and are key to achieving many of the commitments laid out in the NHS Plan. It is, however, important that, as nurses continue to expand their roles to include more technical interventions and care becomes more diverse, they do not lose their holistic approach and devalue the essential caring elements of their role.

> ### Over to you
>
> Read Chapter 7 of the NHS Plan and consider the effect that integration of health and social care may have on the definitions of nursing work and nursing care.

Further details of the plan have been produced, which identify the progress made in respect of the commitments in the plan and set out the priorities for the coming years. The most recent of these is aimed at creating a patient-led service (DOH 2004a). As waiting lists are reducing and access improves, the focus is moving towards greater patient choice, health improvement and the devolution of decision-making.

Following on from this document, the White Paper, *Choosing Health* sets out the planning framework for health and social services for the three years following its publication and covers four national priority areas (DOH 2004b):

- health and well-being of the population;
- long-term conditions;
- access to services;
- patient/user experience.

It sets out Standards for Better Health, which identify the requirements to ensure the provision of safe services of an acceptable quality, which are applicable across the whole range of health care organisations (DOH 2004b). Core and developmental standards are identified and organised within seven domains:

- safety;
- clinical and cost effectiveness;
- governance;
- patient focus;
- accessible and responsive care;
- care environment and amenities;
- public health.

Outcomes for each domain are specified.

The Healthcare Commission (www.healthcarecommission.org.uk) has a responsibility for assessing performance against the standards and taking action to improve performance if a Trust fails to meet the standards. Action taken may be in the form of requiring the Trust to develop proposals for improvement or in exceptional circumstances to take special measures to rectify significant failings.

Reflective activity

One of the commitments in the NHS Plan was to improve access to services. This has been translated into performance targets, which Trusts are measured against. One of these targets is that people presenting at A&E should be seen, treated and be either discharged or admitted to a hospital bed within four hours.

Many Trusts are struggling to meet this target and feel that the targets can sometimes create conflicts in terms of the provision of quality care. Consider how and why such conflict might arise.

Choosing Health

The White Paper *Choosing Health* also specifically addresses the health and well-being of the population, arguing that people need to, and in fact want to, take responsibility for their own health. The paper is based on the principle that people cannot be made to follow a healthy lifestyle, but that the choices they make should be based on reliable information, and they should have the opportunity and support to make healthy choices. The White Paper therefore sets out the support that the government will provide and the action it will take to:

- support informed choice;
- take responsibility for those too young to make informed choices themselves;
- protect the health of the population by preventing people from putting others at risk;
- personalise the support needed to make healthy choices;
- create partnerships with others, e.g. industry, local government, retailers, employers, community and voluntary sector, the media.

It is recognised that health is not solely the responsibility of the health service and, while the health service must place as much priority on promoting health as on treating disease, the health of the population is everyone's responsibility.

Key points | Top tips

- Health care must be seen to be clinically effective and cost efficient.
- It must be accessible to everyone and responsive to individual needs.
- Partnerships between patients and professionals are essential.
- There should be equal priority placed on promoting health and on treating disease.

Quality of care

Plans to address quality and consistency in care were outlined in *A First Class Service* (DOH 1998).

Reflective activity

What does quality of care mean to you?

Below are several different definitions. Which do you feel most reflects your understanding of quality?

1 Meeting or exceeding customer expectations.

2 The totality of features and characteristics of a product that bear on its ability to satisfy a given need (British Standard 4778).

3 Fully meeting the needs of those who need the service most, at the lowest cost to the organisation, within the limits set by higher authorities and purchasers (Ovretveit 1992).

National standards were to be set through the provision of National Service Frameworks and the creation of a National Institute of Clinical Excellence (NICE). In order to ensure that these standards were implemented locally in the delivery of services, a new system called clinical governance would be used to ensure delivery of quality health care.

The third component of this strategy was recognition of the need for lifelong learning by staff to ensure that skills and expertise were maintained and kept pace with changing technology and research. Finally, there were to be three mechanisms to monitor the implementation of clinical governance and national standards. First, there was to be a new statutory body to provide independent scrutiny, to assess local performance and to help address serious problems. Initially, this was called the Commission for Health Improvement, and later, as its remit was expanded, it became the

Healthcare Commission. Second, a national performance framework was introduced in 1999 to assess performance in six key areas:

- health improvement;
- fair access;
- effective delivery of appropriate care;
- efficiency;
- patient/carer experience;
- health outcomes.

Third, a National Survey of Patient/User Experience was to be conducted annually. This multifaceted approach to quality improvement has been further developed and is now firmly embedded in health care services.

National Institute for Clinical Excellence (NICE)

The National Institute for Clinical Excellence (NICE – www.nice.org.uk) was established in 1999 to reduce unnecessary variations in clinical practice and strengthen accountability through the development of national standards. It was recognised that, while research may have shown a new treatment to be effective, the speed at which it was adopted in practice was very variable. For instance, the use of thrombolitic agents in the treatment of myocardial infarction was known to be highly effective, yet this knowledge did not seem to have spread rapidly or evenly. Consequently there were major variations in the management of patients with this condition. Similar variations could be found in relation to other health problems. Knee replacements were known to improve mobility and reduce pain yet, once again, the connection between knowledge and practice was inconsistent even when taking account of different age profiles. Differences in approaches to treatment and care were due to a number of factors, but the vast quantity of information and difficulty in accessing and appraising evidence were major contributory factors.

NICE's role is to bring together clinical evidence and information on the cost effectiveness of treatments and interventions and from this to develop guidelines that are disseminated to all parts of the NHS for implementation.

Some of the guidelines emerging from NICE that tend to attract national publicity are those that relate to the use of new drugs, particularly drugs that are not recommended for use because their effectiveness is not felt to be sufficient to justify the cost. Criticism has been directed at NICE on the grounds that it is not completely impartial because political influences impinge on the recommendations it makes. On the other hand, implementation of many guidelines have cost implications, and all parts of the NHS find budgets severely challenged by the costs associated with providing treatments recommended by NICE.

Viewed purely from a clinical governance perspective, NICE guidelines provide clear evidence about the effectiveness of a growing number of clinical interventions and have enabled practitioners to access information more readily. Previously, each individual practitioner would have needed to carry out a literature search and evaluate evidence from numerous research studies in order to ensure that their practice was evidence based. This process is now carried out systematically by skilled assessors at NICE.

An example of NICE guidance of particular relevance to the provision of nursing care is that relating to pressure ulcer prevention. This guideline identifies the risk factors that predispose an individual to the development of a pressure ulcer and emphasise the need to use clinical judgement in addition to risk assessment scales, which, it recommends, should be used only as an aide mémoire. Most experienced nurses recognise the limitations of risk assessment tools, the majority of which have not been subject to rigorous evaluation of their validity and reliability, but less experienced staff can place too much reliance on such scores. The guideline also recommends that risk assessment should occur within six hours of admission, but identifies that the evidence base for this is less well established.

In respect of preventative action, recommendations are made on positioning of patients, seating and other pressure relieving devices. In the past, items such as synthetic sheepskins, foam rings with a central hole, and water-filled gloves were often used as pressure relieving aids. The guideline clearly states that these should not be used.

This particular guideline was published in 2003 and the recommendations should have been widely implemented. Tissue viability nurses across the UK provide education, advice and support at clinical level, to ensure that members of staff are aware of best practice, and facilitate implementation. However, most will be able to identify examples of outdated practice that they have observed and resource limitations that affect the provision of optimal levels of preventative equipment. Trusts are therefore working towards full implementation of the guideline, which is raising standards, but further progress is needed before the government's vision of consistent implementation across the NHS is fully realised.

Over to you

Visit the NICE website: www.nice.org.uk and look at the range of guidelines available. Choose an example and consider its implementation in an area in which you have worked.

National Service Frameworks (NSFs)

National Service Frameworks (NSFs) set out strategies and standards for specific conditions or areas of care. They identify how services should be organised in order to ensure fair access and quality services. They are developed by bringing together the different professional groups, patients/users and carers, managers, partner organisations, such as social care providers, and the voluntary sector to set long-term strategies. The aims of NSFs are to:

- set national standards with timescales for delivery;
- identify key interventions with the associated evidence base;
- define models of service provision;
- put strategies in place to support implementation.

To date there are NSFs for seven fields of health care:

- coronary heart disease;
- older people;
- cancer;
- paediatric intensive care;
- mental health;
- diabetes;
- long-term conditions.

As with NICE guidance there are frequently cost implications associated with implementation of the frameworks, and the speed of implementation is therefore variable.

Over to you

Clinicians often speak about clinical freedom, i.e. the freedom to make their own decisions about the correct course of action based on their clinical judgement. To what extent do NICE guidelines and NSFs limit clinical freedom? Is this reasonable?

Key points | Top tips

- NICE guidelines and NSFs provide national standards to improve the consistency and quality of care.

Clinical governance

Implementation of continuous quality improvement, and compliance with national standards of excellence, is achieved through a system termed clinical governance, which is defined as 'a framework through which NHS organisations are accountable for continuously improving the quality of their services and safeguarding high standards of care, by creating an environment in which excellence in clinical care will flourish' (DOH 1998).

It is useful to examine some of the key phrases within this definition to understand the changes that clinical governance introduces to the NHS. The first key phrase is *continuous improvement*, which recognises that quality of care is not static and that it is always possible to improve upon what is being done. The definition also includes the concept of *accountability*, recognising that *professional self-regulation* as it stood at the time was not adequate to ensure consistently high standards of care, and that external monitoring was needed. Third, the definition indicates the importance of creating the right *environment* if excellence is to flourish. This environment is one in which there is the ability to recognise where problems exist and ensure that professionals are supported to learn lessons, to improve practice, and to prevent recurrence of similar problems – in other words, to move away from a culture of blame to one of reflection and learning (DOH 1999a).

Some of the main components of clinical governance have implications for nursing care.

Leadership and accountability

Successful clinical governance means that there must be commitment at the level of the Trust Board and clear lines of responsibility for the quality of clinical care. All key groups within an organisation must be committed and involved, as without participation at all levels progress is limited (DOH 1999a). Leaders are needed to provide a vision of the future and motivate people to follow them. They should be able to help staff to translate the vision into practical reality. Leadership in nursing has been the subject of much debate and scrutiny in recent years, and it has been suggested that nursing lacks the leadership necessary to influence health policy (Antrobus and Kitson 1999). At clinical level, it is clear that ward sisters are key to the quality of care the patient receives (RCN 1997). The development and support of clinical leaders was emphasised in *Making a Difference* (DOH 1999b) and makes clear the need for leadership at all levels within nursing. Clinical leadership programmes have been developed nationally to address these concerns both in nursing and across other clinical professions.

A comprehensive programme of quality improvement activity

Standards of care must be monitored and audited within a planned programme for clinical audit, which identifies priorities for audit activity and provides evidence that action has been taken and care improved as a result of the audit activity. Clinical audit can and should occur at a number of different levels. Participation in national comparative audits allows staff to compare their performance with other organisations and national averages. One example of this is the national stroke audit, which examines the management and care of patients admitted to hospital following a stroke. National audits of this type improve consistency of care across the country. Clinical audit may also be performed at Trust level to address an area of concern. Audits of documentation, pressure sores or infection control practices are examples of audits that are often carried out throughout an acute or primary care trust. Audits should also be carried out at ward level to examine and address issues specific to one particular ward/department. Only by continually questioning practice and striving for improvement can nurses truly provide excellence in care and improve the patients' experience. Inherent in standard setting and clinical audit is the requirement to ensure clinical effectiveness and evidence-based practice.

Clinical effectiveness and evidence-based practice

Decisions relating to clinical care must be based on a sound evidence base, including knowledge gained from research. Therefore nurses must keep abreast of research and development in their field of practice and apply it during their clinical decision-making on a day-to-day basis. Access to information and critical appraisal skills are necessary for every nurse wherever they are employed. Patients increasingly have access to information on health issues and treatments through libraries, NHS Direct and the Internet, and should be encouraged to participate in decisions about their care. Staff must therefore be prepared to discuss the rationale supporting the care and treatment they provide. It has been recognised that a national strategy is necessary for the management of information and information technology within the NHS to support the provision of co-ordinated care. There has been considerable progress in this area in recent years, and if the government targets are realised, the NHS will have an extensive electronic patient information system by 2010.

Managing risk

Under clinical governance, clinical risk must be systematically assessed and programmes put into place to reduce that risk. There are risks associated with all aspects of care, and strategies are routinely used to reduce the risks associated with them. Some examples from everyday practice include the risk associated with hospital-acquired infection, the potential to develop pressure sores and risks associated with patient moving and handling. Each Trust has policies to ensure that these risks are managed both at organisational and at individual level. Reducing and managing risk also means that information from clinical incidents, complaints and other patient feedback should be investigated and analysed, and changes put into place to prevent recurrence.

Eliminating poor performance

A number of events reduced public confidence in the NHS, most notably the poor outcomes in paediatric cardiac surgery at Bristol that went unchallenged for a number of years and failures in bone tumour diagnosis in Birmingham. There have also been reports in the national press alleging failures in the provision of basic care, such as the nutrition of patients in hospital and maintenance of personal hygiene. The nurses' code of professional conduct includes a responsibility to act as an advocate for patients and raise concerns about a colleague's professional conduct or performance when necessary (NMC 2002). If concerns are identified at an early stage, individuals can be supported to improve their performance through the provision of support, education or development opportunities. The Nursing and Midwifery Council has a range of procedures to address professional conduct and competency issues. These have been reviewed to modernise and strengthen professional regulation.

Lifelong learning

Professionals need continually to update and develop their practice to keep abreast of technological developments and new research. Nurses have never previously experienced the range of opportunities now available to them, as professional boundaries become more blurred and the potential of nursing is recognised. All nurses should have their own professional development plan (PDP), developed in conjunction with their manager, and access to continuing professional development. Each Trust or organisation will have its own organisational development plan based on the needs of the local community, and individual PDPs will reflect the individual's and the organisation's needs.

Key points | Top tips

- Clinical governance brings together all the elements needed for the provision of safe, effective, high-quality care.
- The Healthcare Commission monitors the effectiveness of clinical governance arrangements within individual Trusts.

Benchmarking

Numerous approaches to the assessment and improvement of quality have been promoted and utilised in the NHS over the last 20 years. These include total quality management, a management philosophy based on the creation of a quality culture, and approaches that focus on systems and processes, such as quality circles, organisational audit, clinical audit and benchmarking. Clinical audit was established in the NHS in the 1980s and remains a central part of clinical governance.

As with clinical audit, benchmarking is a tool that can be used to improve the quality of care by a structured approach to quality assessment and improvement. However, there are some important differences between the two in the way this is achieved.

A benchmark is a standard or point of reference against which some thing or activity may be compared or measured. It therefore follows that the process of benchmarking involves assessment or comparison of performance against a standard or best practice. However, the benchmarking process does not merely measure performance; it identifies how best practice is achieved, and it learns from this, thus raising performance to the levels of the best.

Benchmarking has its origins in industry, where organisations need to maintain a competitive advantage and therefore constantly compare themselves with the market leaders and try to outperform them. The supermarket giants, for example, measure their share of the market, their prices, customer perception of quality, etc. against their competitors, and they identify changes that they can implement in their organisation to achieve better results.

Organisational benchmarking has been defined as: 'the continuous process of measuring products, services, and practices against leaders, allowing identification of demonstrably better practice which will lead to measurable improvements in performance' (Phillips 1995). Benchmarking within industry usually focuses on measuring quantitative outcomes or processes and provides numerical data that can be compared against others. Within the NHS, benchmarking gained some momentum in the 1990s as a means of ensuring value for money and efficiency, and NHS organisations were encouraged to form benchmarking networks. Examples of areas examined within benchmarking include cleaning costs and resources, theatre utilisation and catering. In addition, *The Patient's Charter* (DOH 1991) introduced standards for patient services, and benchmarking against the *Charter* standards was encouraged.

This approach to benchmarking can also be applied to some areas of nursing care. For example, if careful attention is paid to consistent methods of data collection, it is possible to benchmark pressure sore development and management, infection rates and waiting times. Comparison of data from each of these areas will facilitate identification of those with the best results and the factors that contribute to the best outcomes for patients.

However, when seeking to benchmark against the *Charter* standards, it was recognised that some areas that are important to patients, such as privacy and dignity, are more difficult to measure. How do we measure how good we are at addressing a patient's emotional or spiritual needs, our attention to personal hygiene, our communication skills or whether we treat our patients as individuals? Yet these issues are important to the patients themselves and their well-being. A spate of national newspaper articles a few years ago accused hospitals of poor standards of basic care. There were stories of patients being starved because they were not provided with the help they needed to eat and drink and of patients not being offered a bath for several weeks. Reports of the Health Service Commission also drew attention to poor standards of basic care (DOH 1999a). Sadly, complaints managers today would be able to identify examples of patients whose complaints centre around similar aspects of basic nursing care.

Essence of care

The national nursing strategy *Making a Difference* (DOH 1999b) gave a commitment to exploring the potential of benchmarking in improving the quality of the fundamental and essential aspects of care. It cited the experience of paediatric nurses in north-west England who had successfully used benchmarking to improve the care of children in hospital, in areas such as pain assessment, care of adolescents and elective surgery, and suggested that this could be transferred to other areas of care. The importance of basic care to patient well-being and recovery was emphasised and it was reiterated that these are core elements of the nursing function. Here, benchmarking was defined as: 'a process through which best practice is identified and continuous improvement pursued through comparison and sharing'. As a result of this commitment a major project was initiated and came to fruition in the publication of the *Essence of Care* toolkit (DOH 2001b), which contained eight patient-focused benchmarks for health care practitioners:

- continence and bladder and bowel care;
- personal and oral hygiene;
- food and nutrition;
- pressure ulcers;
- privacy and dignity;
- record keeping;
- safety of clients with mental health needs;
- principles of self-care.

Essence of Care differs from many earlier approaches to benchmarking by taking a qualitative rather than a quantitative approach, allowing examination of the quality of the softer aspects of care, which cannot be measured numerically. Large diverse groups of people were brought together to develop each benchmark, including patients, user groups, voluntary organisations, educationalists and researchers as well as clinical professionals. The benchmarks were tested and refined, and consensus agreement was achieved by further consultation. As a result, over 2,000 people contributed to the development of the benchmarks.

A further benchmark covering communication was added in the second edition (DOH 2003). The benchmarks were intended to be applicable across all health care settings, and to all patient groups. Each benchmark contains:

- a *patient focused outcome*, which describes what the benchmark is trying to achieve from the patient's perspective;
- a number of *factors* that contribute to the achievement of the outcome;
- *best practice statements* for each of the factors;

- a *scoring continuum* for each factor to help practitioners identify a score for their own practice and what they are aiming for;
- *indicators* identified by patients and professionals, which may provide evidence that can be assessed to judge whether best practice is being achieved.

They are, therefore, generic in nature, and the evidence required to demonstrate best practice has to be agreed within individual benchmarking groups.

In practice, benchmarking groups come together to examine the extent to which they are achieving best practice, discuss and compare their practice with other group members and learn from each other. They identify changes and improvements that they can make to their practice in order to achieve the best practice statement. From this, an action plan is agreed and reviewed over time to ensure that practice improves and is shared with others. The stages of benchmarking are therefore identified as (DOH 2003):

Stage 1   Agree best practice.

Stage 2   Assess clinical areas against best practice.

Stage 3   Produce and implement an action plan aimed at achieving best practice.

Stage 4   Review progress towards best practice.

Stage 5   Disseminate improvements and review action plan.

Stage 6/1 Agree best practice.

Benchmarking is a cyclical process, facilitating continuous quality improvement. It can be carried out at many different levels within health care settings, and it may involve individuals working together within a ward/department. It may involve wards across a hospital or directorate comparing their practice, or it may involve different NHS Trusts coming together in a benchmarking group. There are numerous articles in the professional press giving accounts of the experiences of benchmarking and the benefits realised. The toolkit can be accessed at www.modern.nhs.uk on the NHS Modernisation Agency website, along with some examples of the practical use of benchmarking with positive outcomes for patients.

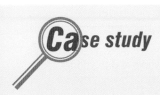

Case study

Edith Brown is a 74-year-old lady admitted to the ward following a stroke. She has a hemiparesis and her speech has been affected. Her husband expressed concern that following her admission she had not had anything to eat or drink for almost a week, and that now that she was allowed to eat and drink freely, she appeared to be eating very little. She needs help with cutting up her food and encouragement to eat, but her husband said that on some occasions when he had visited, he had noticed that her meal tray was collected when very little had been eaten, but that the staff had made no comment. When he had spoken to his wife about it, she had said that she could not manage it on her own and that she did not really like what had been ordered for her. Sister Jones explained to Mr Brown that initially his wife had not been given anything by mouth as the staff were concerned that her swallowing might have been affected, as often happens when someone has a stroke. However, she recognised that there had been a delay in obtaining a speech and language therapy assessment and apologised for this. She said staff did know that Mrs Brown needed help with eating and drinking and she would ensure that staff were reminded of this to prevent similar problems of this kind. Menus were provided so that patients could choose their meals in advance. Mrs Brown should, therefore, be able to choose food she liked so she was surprised that this was an issue. As Sister Jones left Mr Brown, she wondered whether in fact Mrs Brown – who needed help with filling out the menu – had been consulted when the menus were completed for her.

As Sister Jones reflected on what Mr Brown had said, she realised that his concerns were valid and that in fact there had been a written complaint from another patient recently, who had said that the food was unappetising and often cold by the time it was eaten. Sister Jones recognised the importance of nutrition in the patients' recovery, but she also had been unable to solve some of the problems she had identified in respect of nutrition. She had to admit that sometimes mealtimes and nutrition seemed to be less of a priority than activities such as medicine rounds, doctors' ward rounds and wound management. Her ward admitted most of the patients with stroke and had a predominance of elderly patients. Many of these needed help with feeding, and often the number of these outweighed the number of staff available to help with feeding at mealtimes, so people often had to wait and mealtimes were rushed. She also felt that some of the puréed diets looked unappetising, although she had been told they were actually quite tasty. The catering department had recently highlighted the amount of food waste returned to the kitchen from across the hospital and had asked staff to review the ordering of food and completion of menu cards.

As Sister Jones considered the problems, she realised that she needed some help in identifying some possible solutions. She discussed the issues with her senior nurse, who suggested that she might consider starting a benchmarking group and use the *Essence of Care* toolkit as a means of improving practice.

Some of the other wards were also experiencing problems, but there was also some innovative practice in some areas where work had, been done to improve mealtimes for patients.

Read Department of Health (2001b) *Essence of Care*, available at http://www.dh.gov.uk/PublicationsAndStatistics.

Look at the section on nutrition.

What actions could be taken to improve care for patients on Sister Jones' ward?

Compare your ideas with those listed on the Essence of Care web page at http://www.cgsupport.nhs.uk/Resources/Eurekas/Essence_of_Care/default.asp.

Key points Top tips

Benchmarking:

- can be used to examine and improve both the quantifiable and the non-quantifiable aspects of care;
- is consistent with the development of a blame-free culture;
- enables practitioners to compare their practice with others and with the best available evidence;
- encourages user involvement in quality improvement;
- facilitates sharing and helps close the gap between the best and the rest (NHS Plan).

Patient and public involvement

Public dissatisfaction with the NHS has been in part due to a lack of responsiveness to the needs of patients. The NHS provided a service that had to fit all, rather than being flexible enough to respond to changing demands and expectations, and it was recognised that this had to change.

However, this added to the pressure on the NHS created by new medical advances and the aging population. The public was more informed, and expectations were higher, in terms both of quality of care and access to services. While the public are generally supportive of a health service that is free at the point of delivery, they also feel that they have a right to this service, as they contribute through the taxation system.

Modernisation of the NHS therefore sought to address these issues by making the NHS more accountable to the public, by creating a sense of ownership and trust, and by providing a service responsive to the needs of individual patients. Health policies therefore started to emphasise, and continue to endorse, the need for partnerships to be developed between the public and the NHS (DOH 1999c).

Patient and public involvement (PPI) means not only involving people in decisions about their own care but also involving the public in decisions regarding the development and provision of services, 'placing patients at the centre of everything the NHS does'. The aim is to create a 'new model where the voices of the service users act as a powerful lever for change and improvement' (DOH 2001a).

The NHS Plan described a range of initiatives to empower patients, ensure their views are heard and provide protection and rights of redress. These include:

1 Provision of information to empower patients. Patients are to be provided with better information about their condition/treatment through local written information, patient friendly versions of NICE guidelines, NHS Direct information, and expansion of the Expert Patient Programme. There is also a requirement for letters between clinicians about an individual's care to be copied to the patient and easier access by patients to their own records.

2 Greater patient choice. Patients will be able to choose their GP and, in addition, choose when and where they have their hospital treatment. This will be supported by the provision of better information about local services.

3 Patient Advice and Liaison Service (PALS). PALS is a service that was established across the NHS in 2002. It provides information, advice and support to help patients, families and their carers. It can help them to raise and address individual concerns early, before they become more serious, and thereby prevent the need to resort to making a formal complaint. National core standards and an evaluation framework for PALS have been developed to ensure consistency of service provision across the country.

Over to you

Each NHS Trust and Primary Care Trust (PCT) has a PALS. Contact your local PALS and identify some of the issues/themes that are raised by patients in your area.

4 Complaints. The NHS Plan gave a commitment to review the complaints service, to make it more independent and responsive to patients. In addition, an Independent Complaints Advocacy Service (ICAS) is available to provide independent support to people waiting to make a complaint. Written information is available to people wishing to complain and this gives details of how to contact ICAS.

5 Independent patient and public involvement forums have been established for each NHS Trust and PCT. Patients and members of the public from the local community have been recruited to the forums, which have a remit to monitor the quality of local services from the patient's perspective and represent the views of the local community. PPI forums can work together across boundaries where this is appropriate.

6 Accountability. The Health and Social Care Act (2001) places a statutory duty on the NHS to consult patients and the public in

the planning and development of services and when proposing any substantial variation to service. Local Authority Overview and Scrutiny Committees have the ability to scrutinise the NHS and call local NHS chief executives to account.

Theory into Practice

The term 'patient involvement' is often used to denote individual patients' involvement in their care; 'patients are treated as equal partners, listened to and properly informed. Privacy and time for discussion are both required to achieve this', source: www.healthinpartnership.org

'Public involvement' is a corporate responsibility. It includes consulting and involving the public in decisions about service and influences policies, plans and service changes.

Consider the description of patient involvement above and how well this is applied in your experience.

Key points   Top tips

- If the NHS is to be responsive to the needs and expectations of patients and the public, then patients and the public should be involved and consulted in decision-making at all levels.
- To achieve patient and public involvement, consideration must be given to the provision of information, obtaining and acting on feedback, and the provision of opportunities for involvement, at both an individual patient level and collective level with the local population.

National surveys of patient/user experience

A First Class Service (DOH 1998) identified the need for patient/user experience to shape decisions about service and therefore the importance of capturing information about the patients' experience of the NHS as part of the overall assessment of NHS performance.

The first national patient survey was carried out in 2002; it examined inpatient care in acute and specialist Trusts. This was followed in 2003 by the first surveys of Primary Care Trusts (PCTs), A&E departments and outpatient departments. These surveys were repeated in 2004 and surveys of mental health, ambulance Trusts and young patients (acute and specialist inpatients) have also been added. In addition, surveys of stroke patients and patients with coronary heart disease were piloted in 2004.

The surveys are co-ordinated and reported on by the Healthcare Commission and, in the majority of cases, survey 850 people from each Trust. They cover issues that are important for patients and have been developed with the involvement of patients. Results are presented to individual Trusts in a benchmark format that allows comparison with other Trusts. Each Trust is expected to assess the information provided by the surveys and develop action plans to address areas of weakness, and improve their performance. Overall, the findings from the surveys have been very positive in that a large majority of patients rated their care very highly and, in those areas where the surveys have been repeated, access to health care has improved. Some of the areas that have been identified for improvement include:

- information for patients and understanding of explanations given;
- information about medications and their side effects;
- involvement in decisions about care and treatment;
- the hospital environment, including cleanliness and lack of privacy;
- delays on the day of discharge.

Provision of information is an issue that is key to improving the patient's experience, as without appropriate information and understanding a patient will be unable to participate equally in decisions about their care, even if given the opportunity. The information needs of patients vary considerably, as does patients' capacity to understand some of the complexities of treatment options.

It is important, therefore, for the professional to listen to patients and assess carefully the amount of information they wish to have and their level of understanding. Many patients experience stress and anxiety during consultations and may not remember accurately what has been said. They may not like to ask too many questions or, indeed, may forget all their pre-prepared questions once in the consulting room. Patients need time and encouragement to ask questions and voice their fears and anxieties. Patients often also complain that they receive conflicting advice from different professionals. If this occurs they may lose confidence in one or more of the team caring for them. It is therefore very important for the multidisciplinary team to work closely together to reduce the potential for giving conflicting information and to document the information given. Reinforcing verbal information with written information is useful. Communication skills should not be taken for granted, and training in this area must be recognised as a priority for all health care professionals.

- National patient surveys are one method of obtaining patient feedback.
- They should be used alongside other feedback to identify priorities for quality improvement.

Conclusion

Recent health policy has focused on improving the efficiency and effectiveness of health care, ensuring access for all and consistency of standards across the country. This has impacted on approaches to the management and delivery of care and will continue to do so. Performance targets have been set and systems put into place to encourage a culture of continuous quality improvement, although sometimes the drive to improve access can seem to conflict with the drive for improved quality.

Opportunities for professionals have never been greater, but more than ever it is essential that we are able to provide the rationale supporting our care and treatment by the implementation of evidence-based practice. Patient and public expectations of the NHS have increased, and, if public support is to continue, health care has to become an equal partnership between patients and professionals.

RRRRR**Rapid recap**

1 Explain the issue being addressed in the *Choosing Health* White Paper 2004.
2 What are the main components of clinical governance with relation to nursing care?
3 Describe the six stages of benchmarking identified by the Department of Health in 2003.

References

Antrobus, S. and Kitson, A. (1999) 'Nursing leadership: influencing and shaping health policy and nursing practice', *Journal of Advanced Nursing* 29 (3) pp. 746–53.

Department of Health (DOH) (1991) *The Patient's Charter.* London, DOH.

Department of Health (DOH) (1997) *The NHS: Modern and Dependable.* London, DOH.

Department of Health (DOH) (1998) *A First Class Service, Quality in the New NHS.* London, DOH.

Department of Health (DOH) (1999a) *Clinical Governance, Quality in the New NHS.* London, DOH.

Department of Health (DOH) (1999b) *Making a Difference, Strengthening the Nursing, Midwifery and Health Visiting Contribution to Health and Health Care.* London, DOH.

Department of Health (DOH) (1999c) *Patient and Public in the NHS.* London, DOH.

Department of Health (2000) *The NHS Plan. A Plan for Investment. A Plan for Reform.* London, DOH.

Department of Health (DOH) (2001a) *Patient and Public Involvement in the NHS.* London, DOH.

Department of Health (DOH) (2001b) *Essence of Care.* London, DOH.

Department of Health (DOH) (2003) *Essence of Care.* London, DOH.

Department of Health (DOH) (2004a) *NHS Improvement Plan.* London, DOH.

Department of Health (DOH) (2004b) *Choosing Health, Making Healthy Choices Easier.* Public Health White Paper, CM 6374, London, DOH.

Ham, C. (2004) *Health Policy in Britain*, 5th edn. Basingstoke, Palgrave Macmillan.

Nursing and Midwifery Council (NMC) (2002) *Code of Professional Conduct.* London, NMC.

Ovretveit (1992) *Health Service Quality: An Introduction to Quality Methods for Health Services.* London, Blackwell Scientific.

Phillips, S. (1995) 'Benchmarking: providing the direction for excellence', *British Journal of Health Care Management* 1 pp. 705–7.

Royal College of Nursing (RCN) (1997) *RCN Ward Leadership Project – A Journey to Patient Centred Leadership.* London, RCN.

The future for care

Learning outcomes

By the end of this chapter you should be able to:

- summarise the key points about care discussed in this book;
- identify aspects of care that require further investigation;
- identify factors that will influence the future nature and provision of care.

Introduction

Professional nursing in the twenty-first century is a challenging and demanding occupation that is based on the ability to synthesise academic education based on theoretical information with high levels of practical skills. Effective nursing requires the creative adaptation of that synthesis to work with individuals, their families or other groups to which they belong, in ways that enable those people to avoid disease, manage enduring health problems, cope with illness or prepare for death. Nursing work is, therefore, diverse, varying according to the needs of the recipients and the settings in which they encounter the nurse. Such diversity can make it difficult to explain what it is that nurses do or what it is that separates their work from that of other health and social care professionals. There may have been a time when such a lack of clarity did not matter very much, when it could be safely assumed that whatever it was that nurses did was of benefit to their patients. Advances in knowledge, technological development and spiralling costs mean that this is no longer the case. Moreover, social changes have led to both increased expectations of health services and a more critical appraisal of the professionals who provide them. The old assumptions can no longer be relied upon and nursing must make plain its contribution to current health care and how it will evolve to meet future health needs.

Nursing has sought to clarify its contribution to health care in two ways. First, the metaparadigm of nursing identifies the parameters of the profession through four key concepts: *environment*, *health*, *person* and *nursing*. The person is the recipient of nursing activities, that is to say the individual, family or group for whom nursing services are provided. Environment refers to the settings in which those services are delivered, the social environment in which the recipients live or work and the physical and psychological components of each person concerned. Health is determined by what is normal for each individual. It forms the basis of a holistic approach to the provision of nursing itself through systematic assessment, planning, implementation and evaluation. This metaparadigm provides an agreed starting point for nurse theorists to explore further the different ways in which nursing contributes to health care. Each theorist may use particular philosophical ideas or knowledge drawn from other disciplines but the overall intention remains to provide a rational explanation of nursing activity.

A second approach to clarifying the nature of nursing is provided by the concept of care as a central and unifying focus for professional work. This book has enabled you to examine this concept in detail and consider the ways in which care underpins nursing activities in various different settings. This chapter begins by summarising the key points addressed in this book and highlights areas in which the concept of care requires further research with reference to your field of practice. The discussion then goes on to consider how nursing care may develop in future.

Key points about care

This book has emphasised that care is a multifaceted concept that has relational, ontological and intentional dimensions, many of which tend to be taken granted (Edwards 2001). There is thus no single definition of this concept. Nursing research has demonstrated that care provides a focal point for nursing, giving meaning and structure to roles and activities that might otherwise appear disconnected (Leininger 1984). In nursing, care represents a synthesis of two types of knowledge, *knowing how* (theoretical) and *knowing that* (practical), which form a basis for therapeutic nurse–patient relationships and skilled nursing interventions (Benner 1984; Benner *et al.* 1996, 1999). Care is, therefore, the essence, the underlying principle from which nursing activities arise regardless of the form that those activities take. Care is so taken for granted that we frequently lose sight of it completely. Only when it is absent do we realise its power and value. Our patients, the recipients of care, have less difficulty in appreciating the nature and importance of care. For them, the essence of care lies in performance. Technical expertise and clinical competence are important to patients but in their view both must be mediated by interpersonal skills and meaningful evidence of concern (McGee 2000). The true nature of care, therefore, lies in the way in which it is given. *Research is needed in your field of practice to identify those factors that patients experience as care and how these may best be incorporated into everyday work.*

Care arises from respect for others, a belief that people other than the self matter and are of value (Benner and Wrubel 1989). Like care, respect is a concept that is taken for granted and can be interpreted in different ways. For example, it may be equated with good manners, showing courtesy towards others and not talking down to or belittling them (McGee 2000). Peplau (1952) argues that this element of respect is essential to the development of the therapeutic nurse–patient relationship. Failure to treat people courteously at the outset will adversely affect subsequent relations. Alternatively, respect may be regarded as a moral obligation to treat others as equal to the self, as the self would wish to be treated, irrespective of individual differences (McGee 2000). Showing respect in this context is dependent on listening to people, enabling and encouraging them to make their wishes known. McGee (2000) found that patients particularly valued professionals who listened to them and who accepted what they said. Nurses themselves recognised the need to avoid judging people and to accept patients' decisions even if these conflicted with professional advice. Such views indicate that respect is associated not only with concern for others but also with maintaining their dignity, making time for them and supporting them (McGee 2000; Benner and Wrubel 1989).

Respecting and caring for others requires a high level of interpersonal skill and a willingness to engage with other people in ways that move well beyond those of simple courtesy and politeness. Care and respect involve exposure to other people's suffering and distress, their fears and beliefs. Effective care takes account of recipients' beliefs about the cause and nature of changes in their health and how they think these should be managed. Practitioners willing and able to negotiate with patients will find these individuals more receptive to professional expertise and, perhaps, more open about the factors that influence their health. Such negotiation requires new ways of working that help to establish concordance between patients and professionals within the context of culturally diverse populations. *Research is needed in your field of practice to identify the skills required to establish and maintain concordance and the provision of culturally competent nursing care.*

Implicit in the concept of concordance is the intention to discourage dependence on professionals. Effective care is that built on therapeutic relationships that enable patients to take control of their lives in ways that incorporate changes in their health in ways that are consistent with their values and beliefs. Caring is about encouraging independence whenever possible, but at the same time recognising when this cannot be achieved. In promoting independence and concordance, nurses must not increase suffering or distress by demanding that patients take on more than they can cope with. Care requires the provision of physical, psychological and social support to minimise suffering and improve individuals' quality of life when they are unable to do these things for themselves. Care also requires that such support be given to enable people to prepare for death in peace and with dignity (Henderson 1966). *Research is needed in your field of practice to help practitioners strike an effective and compassionate balance between promoting independence and providing practical assistance for patients who are unable to perform activities of daily living without considerable or excessive effort. Even more important is the need to identify and rectify the subtle ways in which patients experience neglect when their needs are downplayed or ignored.*

Finally, nursing must acknowledge that it cannot monopolise care or function in isolation from other professions. Modern health care is a complex activity that requires the expertise of many different professions and their skills. Members of all the health care professions must work together to meet patients' needs. In this multi-professional mode of working the challenge for nurses is to clarify and promote their unique role. Members of other professions may have little understanding of nursing work, and this, coupled with the diversity inherent in nursing itself, can lead them to undervalue the contribution that nurses make to patient care. Consequently, nursing will be regarded in residual terms as those activities that are left over when the entire professional input has been given, useful but of limited relevance to therapeutic intervention. Nurses need to work on promoting understanding of their roles and responsibilities in positive ways that enable them to function as equals within the multi-professional context of modern health care. *Research is needed in your field of practice to establish ways in which this multi-professional working can be enhanced and further developed by enabling colleagues in other professions to gain a clearer understanding of the contribution of nursing to patient care.*

Future care

This book has enabled you to examine nursing care as a holistic, patient-centred undertaking. The provision of such care is a complex task that requires professional education and skill, in the technical, clinical and interpersonal domains, that is introduced in courses leading to registration and then further developed and enhanced through further professional development. Professional education is thus ongoing throughout each practitioner's career, because synthesising knowledge and skills derived from the diverse range of disciplines that inform nursing and applying these to the care of an individual patient in ways that successfully meet that person's health care needs requires considerable intellectual effort that is rooted in a critical approach to practice. This approach is based on three factors: critical analysis, critical action and critical reflexivity. Critical analysis requires an open-minded, questioning attitude that does not accept the status quo without good reason. Critical action requires the ability to evaluate existing practice in the light of new information and the possible introduction of change. Critical reflexivity requires self-awareness and the ability to learn from events (Brechin 2000; Eby 2000).

A critical approach to practice is as much about the type of person the nurse is, how he or she thinks and learns and the level of intellectual ability present to inform the development of practice as it is about the ability to use sophisticated technology or employ specialist clinical knowledge. This is entirely appropriate not only because of the increasing complexity of modern health care but also, and more importantly, because the nurse is a therapeutic agent. In engaging with patients as they experience suffering and distress or feel dehumanised by the impact of the technology that surrounds them, the nurse draws on personal qualities that facilitate understanding of each person's situation. In doing so, nurses are able to presence themselves with patients, to share intimately in the experiences of those patients in ways that transcend the surrounding machinery and trappings of many care environments. This therapeutic use of self is crucial as technology continues to advance (Travelbee 1971). It is surprisingly easy to lose sight of human beings when confronted with the latest fascinating discovery or machine but neither can replace the importance of human contact and compassion both now and in the future.

The nurse's therapeutic use of self is consistent with current trends towards a patient-led health service. This will be characterised by a move away from services dominated by the preoccupations, priorities and concerns of professionals towards those of patients. Professionals will become one of several resources available to patients. Others will include self-care, support from families and friends and self-help networks such as patient organisations (Beasley 2004). Thus professionals will no longer be the final arbiters of health but part of a patient's repertoire for health management.

Implicit in this situation is the need for professionals to adopt new, patient-centred ways of working that inspire and promote confidence. Within the NHS, nurse leaders have already begun to identify ways in which nursing roles will change for the benefit of patients (see Table 11.1) and the NHS Modernisation Agency has identified what it calls ten high-impact factors that will facilitate better, patient-focused service provision (see Table 11.2). In addition the Agency has identified eleven clinical fields in which specific improvements will be introduced (see Table 11.3). Alongside such development must be attention to standards that ensure the application of best practice by drawing on resources such as the National Institute for Clinical Excellence (www.nice.org.uk) and the use of clinical governance procedures. Patients, too, will have to learn new ways of dealing with their health problems, by becoming better informed about the factors that affect their health and more independent in the care of minor ailments. Such developments will require extensive public education and a major cultural shift away from dependence on professionals.

Table 11.1 Ten key roles for nurses

Suitably prepared nurses should be able to

1 order diagnostic tests for patients, for example X-rays, rather than have patients wait to see a doctor;

2 make and receive referrals directly without having to seek agreement or a countersignature from a doctor;

3 admit and discharge patients with specific conditions and within agreed protocols;

4 manage patient caseloads in relation to specific conditions such as diabetes;

5 provide nurse-led clinics in relation to specific conditions and within agreed protocols;

6 prescribe medicines and treatments;

7 perform resuscitation procedures;

8 perform minor surgery and other procedures for outpatients;

9 provide triage for patients and direct them to the most appropriate health professional;

10 provide leadership in local health services.

Source: DOH (2002)

Table 11.2 Ten high-impact changes that improve health care

1   providing surgery on a day-care basis whenever possible to increase the number of hospital beds available;
2   improving access to key diagnostic tests to reduce unnecessary waiting time;
3   managing variation in patient discharge to reduce length of stay in hospital;
4   managing variation in patient admissions to reduce the number of operations cancelled for non-clinical reasons;
5   avoiding unnecessary follow-up appointments;
6   increasing the reliability of the performance of therapeutic interventions;
7   applying a systematic approach to care for people with long-term conditions;
8   improving patient access to reduce queues;
9   identifying bottlenecks in service provision and devising ways of reducing these;
10 redesigning and extending professional and other roles in line with more efficient patient pathways.

Source: www.content.modern.nhs.uk

Table 11.3 Clinical themes for modernisation

Cancer care	ENT/audiology
Heart disease	Dentistry
Diabetes	Neurology
Orthopaedics	Urology
Dermatology	Plastic surgery
General surgery	

Source: www.content.modern.nhs.uk

In all of this it is important for professionals to ensure that, even if they cannot assist patients in solving their health problems, they at the very least will do no harm. Current campaigns such as that aimed at preventing the spread of hospital-acquired infections and efforts to reach out to underserved and marginalised social groups provide instructive examples of the ways in which harm has been done through neglect or ignorance. Future care providers must be vigilant in avoiding such errors and seek to do their best in providing humane, thoughtful and compassionate care to patients.

References

Beasley, C. (2004) *Leading Together*. Paper presented at the Chief Nursing Officer's Conference and available at www.dh.gov.uk.

Benner, P. (1984) *From Novice to Expert. Excellence and Power in Clinical Nursing Practice*. Menlo Park CA, Addison-Wesley.

Benner, P. and Wrubel, J. (1989) *The Primacy of Caring. Stress and Coping in Health and Illness*. Menlo Park CA, Addison-Wesley.

Benner, P., Tanner, C. and Chesla, C. (1996) *Expertise in Nursing Practice. Caring, Clinical Judgement and Ethics*. New York, Springer Publishing Company.

Benner, P., Hooper-Kyriakidis, P. and Stannard, D. (1999) *Clinical Wisdom and Interventions in Critical Care: A Thinking-in-action Approach*. Philadelphia PA, W. B. Saunders.

Brechin, A. (2000) 'Introducing critical practice', Chapter 2 in A. Brechin, H. Brown and M. Eby (eds) *Critical Practice in Health and Social Care*. Buckingham, Open University Press, pp. 25–47.

Department of Health (DOH) (2002) *Developing Key Roles for Nurses and Midwives: A Guide for Managers*. London, DOH.

Eby, M. (2000) 'Understanding professional development', Chapter 3 in A. Brechin, H. Brown and M. Eby (eds) *Critical Practice in Health and Social Care*, Buckingham, Open University Press, pp. 48–70.

Edwards, S. D. (2001) *Philosophy of Nursing. An Introduction*. Houndmills, Basingstoke, Palgrave.

Henderson, V. (1966) *The Nature of Nursing*. New York, Macmillan.

Leininger, M. (1984) *Care: the Essence of Nursing and Healthcare*. Detroit IL, Wayne State University Press.

McGee, P. (2000) *Culturally-sensitive Nursing: A Critique*. Unpublished PhD thesis. Birmingham, University of Central England.

Peplau, H. (1952) *Interpersonal Relations in Nursing*, New York, G. P. Putnam.

Travelbee, J. (1971) *Interpersonal Aspects of Nursing*. Philadelphia PA, F. A. Davis.

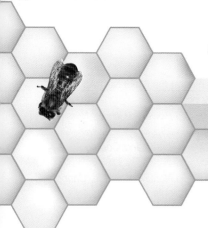

Appendix 1

Summary of nursing theories used in this text

The boxes below provide a summary of the main nursing theories discussed in this book. They help to show the differences and similarities between the different theorists and, in particular, highlight the degree of emphasis that each affords the four elements of the metaparadigm for nursing.

Patricia Benner

Reference

Benner, P. (1984) *From Novice to Expert. Excellence and Power in Clinical Nursing Practice*. Menlo Park CA, Addison Wesley.

Person

The person is a self-interpreting being who is a unified whole. There is no division between mind and body and therefore intelligence and practical skill are embodied attributes that facilitate interpretation and understanding of the world.

Health

Well-being and being ill are interpretations of experiences by the person concerned. Health is more than the absence of disease and may co-exist with disease or disability.

Environment

The environment is the situation with which the person is currently interacting and therefore interpreting.

Nursing

Nursing is primarily about providing care. In learning to care, the nurse passes through five stages of development: novice, advanced beginner, competent, proficient and expert. The practice of nursing draws together theoretical and practical knowledge. There are seven domains of practical knowledge: (1) the helping role; (2) the teaching/coaching function; (3) the diagnostic and patient monitoring function; (4) effective management of rapidly changing situations; (5) administering and monitoring of therapeutic interventions and regimens; (6) monitoring and ensuring the quality of health care practices; (7) organisational and work-role competences.

Madeleine Leininger

Reference

Leininger, M. and McFarland, M. (2002) *Transcultural Nursing: Concepts, Theories, Research and Practice*, 3rd edn. New York, McGraw Hill.

Person

The person is a cultural being who shares learned and transmitted values, beliefs and norms with a particular group. These values, beliefs and norms inform decision-making and daily living. Members of all cultures engage in care. Care is thus a universal phenomenon, but in each culture ideas about what constitutes care vary. Traditional/folk care is culturally defined and practised and directed towards helping, supporting or improving health.

Health

Health is culturally defined and valued.

Environment

The environment can be an event, situation, place or experience that has cultural meaning or significance.

Nursing

Nursing is a professional, learned and humanistic art and science that is directed towards care and provides support and facilitation that enables individuals to maintain or regain their health or prepare for death in ways that are meaningful and culturally appropriate. There are three types of nursing intervention: (1) *culture care preservation* refers to activities intended to help people maintain or regain their health in ways that are wholly consistent with their cultural values and beliefs; (2) *culture care accommodation* activities help patients to adapt to meet the challenges posed by changes in their health in culturally acceptable ways; (3) *culture care repatterning* refers to nursing interventions that facilitate change. The goal of nursing is to provide culturally congruent care to patients.

Myra Levine

Reference

Levine, M. (1967) 'The four conservation principles of nursing', *Nursing Forum* 6 p. 45.

Person

The person is a holistic being composed of integrated systems and dependent on relationships with others for survival. Each person is in a constant state of change. Change occurs through adaptation. The end product of adaptation is *conservation* of (1) energy; (2) structural integrity; (3) personal integrity; (4) social integrity.

Health

Health is a changing state defined by what is considered normal by the social group to which the person belongs. Health is more than the absence of disease or illness. Achieving health requires adaptation, by the person, in terms of conservation of energy, structural integrity, personal integrity and social integrity.

Environment

The internal environment is focused on homoeostasis, a state of energy sparing that facilitates the regulation of the internal environment through physiological and psychological systems. The external environment constantly challenges the internal environment through the senses, communication and other factors.

Nursing

Nursing is a human interaction in which the nurse assists the, individual to adapt positively and achieve conservation. Assessment depends on interviewing skills and observation as the basis for *trophicognosis*, nursing judgement.

Betty Neuman

Reference

Neuman, B. and Fawcett, J. (2002) *The Neuman Systems Model*. Upper Saddle River NJ, Prentice Hall.

Person

The person is an individual or group and is represented as a system, bounded by lines of defence, that is, in constant interaction with the environment and thus in a constant state of change. The individual or group is viewed holistically with physiological, psychological, sociocultural, developmental and spiritual components. The person experiences stressors that are generated by stimuli that arise from the interactions of the person's system with the environment. Adaptation to stressors in the internal or external environments is referred to as reconstitution.

Health

Wellness exists when the various components in the person are in a state of harmony. Health and illness are viewed as opposites on a continuum. Health occurs when the total needs of the person's system are being met.

Environment

Both the internal and external environments can create stressors, which may be physiological, psychological, sociocultural or developmental in origin and can undermine the individual's lines of defence. There is also a created environment, which is developed unconsciously and which allows the individual to reduce stress.

Nursing

Nursing is holistic and concerned with the person's response to stressors. Nursing interventions are intended to help the person strengthen or restore the lines of defence. There are three types of nursing intervention: (1) *primary* intervention is carried out when a stressor is suspected or identified but the person has not yet reacted; (2) *secondary* intervention is provided after the person has reacted to a stressor to stabilise the lines of defence; (3) *tertiary* intervention is provided to help the person readjust once the secondary intervention has been effective.

Florence Nightingale

Reference

Nightingale, F. (1860/1969) *Notes on Nursing: What It Is and What It Is Not.* New York, Dover Publications.

Person

The person is the passive recipient of the nurse's care, which allows Nature to promote healing and recovery.

Health

Health is being well, not being ill. Disease is a reparative process that is affected by the environment, which causes illness and can affect the progress of an illness or disease.

Environment

The environment is everything that is external to the person. The environment can affect health through factors such as poor ventilation, noise, dirt and poor lighting.

Nursing

The nurse is first of all a woman, and every woman will at some time be responsible for the health of others. The goal of nursing is to promote the optimum conditions for Nature to effect recovery from illness.

Dorothea Orem

Reference

Orem, D. (2001) *Nursing: Concepts of Practice*, 6th edn, St Louis MO, C. V. Mosby.

Person

The person is an individual or group who when mature is capable of and motivated towards self-care, which is defined in terms of universal, developmental and health deviation requisites. Self-care is linked to the individual's stage of development, capability and the adequacy with which he or she can perform. Deficiencies in one or more of these three categories results in a self-care deficit.

Health
Health is a state of sound physical and mental functioning.

Environment
The physical environment includes all aspects of the world that are external to the person, such as objects, animals, insects, chemicals, gases, etc. The socioeconomic environment comprises family, work, culture, leisure and available resources. The community environment is concerned with society as a whole and the services or resources that it provides.

Nursing
The nurse aims to facilitate self-care by enabling the patient to achieve independence. The nurse identifies the patient's present and future self-care demands and factors that may help or hinder the performance of self-care. The nurse selects interventions from three categories of activity that will promote self-care: (1) *wholly compensating* for the patient's self-care deficiencies; (2) *partially compensating* for the patient's self-care deficiencies; (3) *providing support and education* that facilitate self-care.

Hildegard Peplau

Reference
Peplau, H. (1952) *Interpersonal Relations in Nursing*, New York, G. P. Putnam.

Person
The person is an individual with physical, social and, especially, psychological needs that generate tension to which each individual reacts in a different way that is evident in his/her behaviour. Each individual is capable of growing and changing.

Health
Health is a dynamic concept in which there is personal growth. Health is always changing and can fail for all sorts of reasons that include lack of resources, failure on the part of health professionals to organise themselves properly or instances where the patient has been ill so long that he or she has forgotten what it is to be well. Illness is a potential learning experience.

Environment
The environment is defined in sociocultural terms as forces such as customs, social mores and beliefs that impact on interpersonal interactions.

Nursing

Nursing is a psychodynamic process between the patient and the nurse in which both parties can learn from each other. The nurse–patient relationship has four phases: orientation, identification, exploitation and resolution. The nurse may adopt any or all of six identified roles: stranger, resource, teacher, leader, counsellor or surrogate.

Nancy Roper, Winifred Logan and Alison Tierney

Reference

Roper, N., Logan, W. and Tierney, A. (2000) *The Roper-Logan-Tierney Model of Nursing: Based on Activities of Living*. Edinburgh, Churchill Livingstone.

Person

The person is an individual who pursues the complex process of living in a unique manner through the activities of living. These activities are influenced by the person's place on the lifespan continuum, and by physical, psychological, sociocultural, environmental and politico-economic factors.

Health

Health and illness are viewed on a continuum but can co-exist. A person can feel healthy even though disease or disability are present. Health is affected by physical, psychological, sociocultural, environmental and politico-economic factors.

Environment

The environment is seen principally in terms of its influence on the individual's ability to perform the activities of living. The scope of this influence is very wide and can include global factors such as food supplies, going into hospital and the effects of illness on an individual's routine.

Nursing

The goal of nursing is to identify actual and potential problems and to provide interventions that promote or restore health or enable someone to have a peaceful death.

Callista Roy

Reference

Roy, C. and Andrews, H. (1999) *The Roy Adaptation Model*, Stamford CN, Appleton Lange.

Person

The person is a bio-psycho-social being in constant interaction with the environment and capable of adaptation in response to stimuli which may be internal or external in origin. Adaptation is controlled by two mechanisms: (1) the *regulator* system deals with unconscious activity such as physiological responses; (2) the *cognator* system deals with conscious activity such as learning and making decisions. The person has *four adaptive modes*: (1) physiological; (2) self-concept; (3) role concept; (4) interdependence.

Health

Health is an adaptive state, the result of coping effectively with the environment. Health and ill health are an inevitable part of a person's life.

Environment

The internal physiological and psychological environments produce stimuli to which the individual has to respond and adapt. The external physical and social environments produce stimuli to which the individual has to respond and adapt.

Nursing

Nursing is a practical activity directed towards the promotion of positive adaptation in the four adaptive modes as a means of either improving health or enabling someone to die with dignity.

Joyce Travelbee

Reference

Travelbee, J. (1971) *Interpersonal Aspects of Nursing*. Philadelphia PA, F. A. Davis.

Person

The person is a human being. Both patients and nurses are human beings, unique individuals who are constantly changing and evolving. The nurse is a human being who has specialised knowledge that can be used to prevent illness or to care for the sick or the dying.

Health

Health has two dimensions: (1) *subjective* refers to the patient's views of his/her state of health; (2) *objective* refers to the absence of disease/disability as confirmed by laboratory tests, or by psychological or spiritual assessments. Illness can be subjective or objective in origin and is associated with pain, suffering, hope and hopelessness.

Environment

The environment is not specifically defined.

Nursing

Nursing is an interpersonal process in which the nurse consciously uses the self as a means of providing appropriate interventions.

Jean Watson

Reference

Watson, J. (1999) *Nursing, Human Science and Human Care. A Theory of Nursing*. Boston MA, Jones and Bartlett Publishers and National League for Nursing.

Person

The person is primarily a spiritual being who has mental, physical and sociocultural dimensions that give rise to a hierarchy of needs. Basic needs such as food and breathing must be attended to before higher order ones such as self-actualisation.

Health

Health is a state of unity and harmony between the mind, body and spirit. Illness is a state rather than the presence of disease. Illness can occur as the result of spiritual distress.

Environment

The environment can be a specific situation in the physical or social world or viewed in terms of social interactions.

Nursing

Care is a core component of nursing, and caring is expressed in the transpersonal caring relationship. Nurses have a moral commitment to care. Caring is based on *ten carative factors*, which are: (1) humanistic and altruistic values; (2) instilling hope; (3) sensitivity to self and others; (4) development of trust between nurse and patient; (5) sharing and accepting that feelings about a situation may differ; (6) a problem-solving approach;
(7) promoting patients' independence through education; (8) providing support and protection and promoting well-being; (9) recognising patients' needs; (10) using situations to achieve a deeper understanding of aspects of care or care giving.

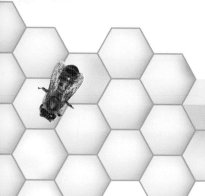

Appendix 2

Rapid recap – answers

Chapter 1

1   **The three elements required in the critical approach to practice are critical analysis, critical action and critical reflexivity.**

2   **The key skills needed for each element are:**
    (i)   for critical analysis: the ability to analyse and evaluate new information, and to make decisions about the extent to which such information is credible and likely to make a useful contribution to practice;
    (ii) for critical action: the ability to identify the criteria for success and the likely obstacles, planning the introduction of change and evaluating progress;
    (iii) for critical reflexivity: the development of self-awareness through the use of reflective skills by each practitioner.

3   **Intentional, relational and ontological aspects of care are explained as follows:**
    (i)   intentional care: care that is consciously directed towards others;
    (ii) relational care: care that helps, supports or facilitates another individual;
    (iii) ontological care: care that is part of our experience of being in the world, i.e. care is an integral part of what it is to be a human being.

4   **The three factors that influence nursing care are social factors, international factors and nursing itself.**

    Societal changes have meant that professionals now have a much greater responsibility to explain to patients the courses of action available and to help individuals to make informed and appropriate choices that suit their circumstances. International factors have influenced both UK law and the practice of nursing. Nursing practice itself has led to revisions in such documents as the Code of Professional Conduct that have reflected the impact of the human rights legislation and the changes that have taken place in society during the preceding decade.

Chapter 2

1   **Nurses should adopt a different nursing approach according to the needs of each patient group because patient groups differ in terms of both their conditions and the degree of nursing interventions required. Furthermore, thinking about the particular patient groups helps us to ensure that we see them more clearly as people like ourselves and leads us into considering how they may experience the care we provide.**

2   **We can consider how patients might experience care by relying on how people react to our interventions, what they tell us about these reactions and what we ourselves have learned as recipients of care from others.**

3   **The four aspects of care that patients perceive as indicators of good care from nurses are:**
    - interpersonal skills
    - showing concern
    - practical help
    - performance.

4   **The aspects of nursing care that patients most commonly find lacking are those relating to basic nursing care, that is, care that is fundamental to individual well-being,**

such as washing oneself, performing mouth care, eating, drinking, moving around and breathing easily.

5 When monitoring patient goals the nurse must continually consider that they must be specific, measurable, realistic, time limited and individualised.

Chapter 3

1 The nursing process comprises four phases: assessment, planning, implementation and evaluation.

2 Successful completion of an assessment is dependent on three factors:

(i) The nurse must possess interpersonal skills that can be used constructively to explore the patient's problems and build the foundations of a subsequent therapeutic relationship.

(ii) The patient must be willing to engage in the assessment by contributing information and by working with the nurse.

(iii) The nurse requires an assessment framework that guides the gathering and interpretation of information in ways that facilitate the formulation of accurate diagnoses.

3 The five elements that form the basis of the Roper, Logan and Tierney model of assessment are:

(i) individuality in living – no two people are exactly alike either as people or in the ways in which they live their lives;

(ii) activities of living that all individuals perform in a unique way and that may be affected by a change in health status that may arise because of the third element;

(iii) biological, psychological, sociocultural, politico-economic or environmental factors;

(iv) the individual's age and stage of development with regard to each activity;

(v) the person's level of independence or dependence with regard to each activity.

4 A nursing diagnosis is a professional judgement, based on the nurse's understanding of the patient's situation, about factors that are within the sphere of nursing work and expressed in a way that is meaningful to other nurses and, where appropriate, to members of other disciplines.

Chapter 4

1 Direct care is care given by a nurse to an individual patient. Washing a patient, performing mouth care, administering medication and recording blood pressure are all examples of direct care.

2 Indirect care is care provided by nurses who have no direct contact with the patient. Educating staff, writing standards and providing clinical supervision are all examples of indirect care.

3 Travelbee's (1971) therapeutic use of self referred to the ways in which nurses can consciously use their own personal attributes and experience to engage with and support patients.

4 The meaning of the terms nurse consultant, modern matron and specialist nurse are as follows:

● A nurse consultant provides clinical leadership and expertise in a specific field of practice.

● A modern matron provides a point of contact for patients and relatives and leadership in ensuring that standards of service provision are met.

● A specialist nurse is one who has undertaken post-registration education to develop a deeper knowledge base and skill in relation to a specific field of care, for example nutrition or tissue viability.

5 Clinical practice benchmarking is a cyclical process that involves:

● identifying areas of practice where standards are needed;

● evaluation of the evidence that underpins good practice;

● grading good practice;

● comparing practice between teams in the same field;

● setting, monitoring and reviewing standards.

Chapter 5

1 The main focus of primary care is to enable people to improve or maintain their health, to diagnose and treat a range of conditions and illness and to refer patients, where necessary, to other sources of help in secondary care.

2 Long-term health conditions affect patients as they present enduring or permanent challenges to an individual's internal environment and to that person's ability to interact with the social or physical world outside the self.

3 Community matrons are experienced, skilled nurses. Their role is to use case management techniques to help patients who depend on health service support because they have one or more long-term conditions. The aim is to help them manage their condition as independently as possible, prevent unnecessary admissions to hospital and, when admissions are essential, reduce the length of the patient's stay. Community matrons also work to provide better communication between primary and secondary service providers to promote seamless care. Community matrons are responsible for identifying and monitoring high-risk patients and, when they are admitted to hospital, instigating an in-reach programme. This means that the community matron will work with hospital staff to plan discharge and incorporate recommended changes into the patient's long-term management plan.

4 The Healthcare Commission is concerned with standards in health care. The Commission inspects and assesses the performance of organisations that provide health care both in the NHS and in the independent sector, in both secondary and primary care settings. The assessment is based around specific targets that each type of organisation is expected to achieve and the standard required.

Chapter 6

1 Culture is important in health care because:
   - it influences what people think about health and illness and their views about care;
   - nurses have a professional responsibility to show respect for cultural values and beliefs and to ensure that everyone receives appropriate care;
   - current health service reforms aim to widen access to care, making services more appropriate to the cultural and other needs of local populations.

2 The advantages and disadvantages of using existing nursing tools to assess cultural issues in nursing care are as follows:
   - Advantages: nurses are more likely to remember cultural issues, and using what is already in place can help to identify a range of culturally diverse issues, for example in relation to food, communication and other factors.
   - Disadvantages: existing tools may not allow for sufficient depth, and some important factors may be omitted.

3 The advantages and disadvantages of using specific tools to assess cultural issues in nursing care are:
   - Advantages: specialist tools may help to develop a more detailed and comprehensive picture.
   - Disadvantages: specialist tools may be very lengthy and complex. Nurses may forget or not have time to do an additional assessment.

4 Cultural competence refers to the ability of an individual to work effectively within the cultural context of another person. It is a continuous process of learning, reflecting and acting in ways that incorporate cultural issues into care.

5 Concordance means negotiating with the patient about the nature and suitability of the care and treatment available to establish a mutually agreed plan of action based on the individual's circumstances. It is the opposite of compliance in which professionals tell patients what to do.

Chapter 7

1   **The aim of the expert patient scheme is intended to complement professional roles by helping those with long-term conditions to:**

- become better informed about their health problems;
- manage their health problems more independently;
- engage in self-help and self-care.

2   **Two ways in which the Internet may be used to share good practice are:**

- through work-based intranets, professional forums such as those provided by the Royal College of Nursing and discussion networks;
- through clinical practice benchmarking in identifying standards and comparing practice.

3   **The key points to remember in evaluating websites for health care are:**

- to keep an open mind and be willing to discuss new ideas with the patient;
- to use evaluative skills to consider:
  - suitability and appropriateness for patients and colleagues;
  - accuracy and currency of the content;
  - ownership of the site and intended aims or function;
  - user-friendliness and security;
  - relevance to UK health care practice.

4   **The two types of nursing knowledge that have been outlined in this chapter are 'knowing that' and 'knowing how':**

- 'Knowing that' is the knowledge that develops over time as a result of experience and the performance of nursing work and that cannot always be explained theoretically.
- 'Knowing how' is the theoretical knowledge that is obtained from formal sources such as books and courses and that explains, describes or predicts events in nursing.

5   **One of the advantages of involving patients in designing a website is the insight that patients' experiences can provide into the types of information that other patients will find most useful and how that information can best be presented. In addition, involving patients will improve the quality of** information available and challenge stereotypical thinking.

Chapter 8

1   **The three main forms of skill mix are:**

(i)   mix of skills across different health disciplines involved in delivering a service;

(ii)   mix of skills held within a particular discipline (including trained staff and associated support staff);

(iii)   mix of skills held by an individual.

2   **A team is a group of people who share common objectives and who need to work together to achieve these. Three types of need are present in every team are:**

- individual
- group
- task.

3   **The four stages of team development are:**

Stage 1   Orientation, testing and dependency stage. During this stage, individual needs are dominant as individuals try to find out whether their personal needs will be met.

Stage 2   Intra-conflict stage. During this stage the emphasis is on meeting team and individual needs. Team needs include such things as ground rules, team structure and modes of communicating. Little work gets done in either this or the previous stage.

Stage 3   Team cohesion. In this stage a bit more time is spent on the task, but the bulk of the time is spent on team needs, while less time is spent on individual needs.

Stage 4   Problem solving and interdependence. During this stage approximately equal amounts of time are spent on individual, team and task needs.

4   **There are a number of factors that have been found to help in the development of multidisciplinary teams. These include:**

- personal commitment
- sharing a common goal
- clarity of roles
- good lines of communication
- institutional support
- leadership.

5   **Three factors that can inhibit interprofessional teamwork are:**

(i)   Attitudes of team members. If one or more of the team members is unconvinced about the advantages of multidisciplinary working, or even opposed to this, they can severely affect the co-ordination of care delivery.

(ii)   Time and resource constraints. If there are staff shortages it can prove difficult to support interprofessional activities that are time consuming. Organising and attending meetings when all members can be available can be problematic, particularly when 'getting people together' takes staff away from their care delivery work. Accommodation for meetings may be limited, and geographical distance between staff can add to the pressures of everyday working. Access to evidence to underpin practice decisions may also be limited by the availability of information technology and library resources.

(iii)   The differing professional bodies. Health care professionals must work within their accountability and legal framework. When professionals work collaboratively they must constantly review whether they are acting within the 'rule of law' and whether, if they perform a task previously done by another health care professional, this is done to the same standard (the 'rule of negligence').

Chapter 9

1   **The seven domains of nursing identified by Benner are:**

- the helping role;
- the teaching/coaching function;
- the diagnostic and patient monitoring function;
- the effective management of rapidly changing situations;
- administering and monitoring therapeutic interventions or regimens;
- monitoring and ensuring the quality of health care practice;
- organisational and work role competencies.

2   **Students can learn from expert nurses by watching them when they deliver care, by** questioning them about their care decisions and reflecting on how they approach their nursing care.

3   **Clinical scholarship means having a willingness to scrutinise practice, challenging the theories and practice that have already been learnt, and looking for better ways of doing things.**

4   **Evidence-based practice involves basing a practice decision on the best available evidence. This may be in the form of relevant research literature or expert opinion. The object is to weigh up all of the available evidence available, compare this to the practice that currently exists and decide how the current practice could change to improve the care that is being provided.**

5   **Barriers to the implementation of evidence-based practice are:**

- Everyday work demands in practice areas.
- Emphasis on the caring aspects of nursing to the detriment of the scientific aspects.
- Limited useful texts and electronic sources to support practice.
- Lack of tine for health care staff to keep abreast of new information by reading journals and accessing other external evidence.
- Insufficient time or resources to undertake original research.

Chapter 10

1   **The *Choosing Health* White Paper 2004 recognises that people need, and want, to take responsibility for their own health. The White Paper sets out the support that the government will provide and the action it will take to:**

- support informed choice;
- take responsibility for those too young to make informed choices themselves;
- protect the health of the population by preventing people from putting others at risk;
- personalise the support needed to make healthy choices;

- create partnerships with others, e.g. industry, local government, retailers, employers, community and voluntary sector, the media.

2   The main components of clinical governance with relation to nursing care are:

- leadership and accountability;
- a comprehensive programme of quality improvement activity;
- clinical effectiveness and evidence-based practice;
- managing risk;
- eliminating poor performance;
- lifelong learning.

3   The six stages of benchmarking identified by the Department of Health in 2003 are:

Stage 1   Agree best practice.

Stage 2   Assess clinical areas against best practice.

Stage 3   Produce and implement an action plan aimed at achieving best practice.

Stage 4   Review progress towards best practice.

Stage 5   Disseminate improvements and review action plan.

Stage 6/1 Agree best practice.

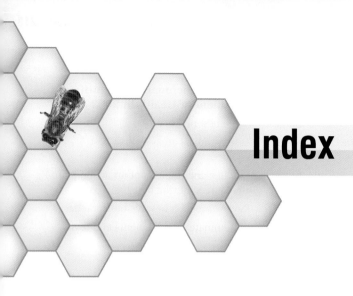

Index